Healthcare and Spirituality

Stephen P Kliewer D.Min.

Executive Director
Wallowa Valley Center for Wellness
Assistant Professor
Department of Family Medicine
Oregon Health & Science University

and

John Saultz MD

Professor and Chairman
Department of Family Medicine
Oregon Health & Science University

Radcliffe Publishing
Oxford • Seattle

Radcliffe Publishing Ltd
18 Marcham Road
Abingdon
Oxon OX14 1AA
United Kingdom

www.radcliffe-oxford.com
Electronic catalogue and worldwide online ordering facility.

British Library Cataloguing in Publication Data

A catalogue record for this book is available from the British Library.

ISBN 1 85775 622 3

Typeset by Advance Typesetting Ltd, Oxford, UK
Printed and bound by TJ International Ltd, Padstow, Cornwall, UK

Contents

Preface   iv

About the authors   vi

1 Healing, cure, and the whole person   1

2 Toward a model of integration   24

3 Exploring spirituality   46

4 The impact of spirituality   63

5 The culture of one   84

6 The objectives of integrating spirituality and medicine   109

7 First steps, gathering information   126

8 Spiritual assessment   147

9 Spiritual interventions   166

Epilogue   191

Appendix A: Active listening skills   192

Appendix B: The Spiritual Involvement and Beliefs Scale   204

Appendix C: Sample meditations, writing exercises, and drawing exercises   208

Appendix D: Suggested further reading   212

Index   215

Preface

We are now halfway through the first decade of the twenty-first century and medicine is experiencing a profound transition. Scientific advances have empowered physicians with tools unimaginable only a generation ago and life expectancy is increasing globally. The human genome has been decoded, promising even more rapid technical advancement in the years to come. But there is a deep sense of discontent with healthcare. Rapidly increasing costs have made basic services inaccessible to millions of people. As medicine has become more technically sophisticated, both patients and physicians are experiencing a loss of the personal healing touch, which has been such an important fundamental of the doctor–patient relationship. Reports have documented an alarming rate of error in healthcare systems, errors that harm patients and undermine trust. Increasingly disillusioned by the allopathic model of medicine, and feeling distanced from their healers, patients have turned more frequently to alternative models of healthcare, and to resources such as spirituality.

Many authors view the problems of uncontrolled cost, poor access, erosion of trust, and lack of safety as evidence that our approach to healthcare requires radical reform. Nowhere are these problems more urgent than in the delivery of basic primary care services at the community level. Several medical specialties have undertaken extensive reviews of the current model of care and are working to address these problems. But there is a clear and widening gulf between what patients want from healthcare and what the healthcare system can provide. Physicians tend to view healthcare as a biologic process in which patient problems are best understood as mechanical dysfunction of one or more body systems. But patients visit the physician with a wide array of problems, many of which cannot be understood on the basis of biology alone.

Increasingly, the biomedical model of healthcare is proving incapable of meeting the needs of those we seek to serve. The specialty of family medicine has addressed this problem over the past 35 years by broadening the focus of attention to address psychological, social, family, and community issues as well as basic biologic diagnosis in the process of caring for patients. Described by some authors as a 'biopsychosocial model' and by others as 'contextual care,' the new model seeks to individualize care by addressing patient problems rather than only their medical diagnoses as the focus of care.

Into this environment, we offer this introductory textbook, dedicated to a systems approach with emphasis on also integrating spiritual issues into the process of healthcare. We believe that most people consider themselves to be spiritual beings and approach spiritual growth across an incredible spectrum of faith systems from traditional religious denominations to new-age spirituality. Traditional Western medicine has generally considered the spiritual to be outside of the physician's focus of attention. Chapters 1 and 2 describe how this came to be and why such restrictions limit our ability to help many of our patients. We then seek in the remaining chapters to create a framework for talking about spiritual issues with patients. When is it appropriate for physicians to assess spiritual health in the context of delivering healthcare? How can we raise these issues with patients without disrupting the foundation of trust in the doctor–patient relationship? How can we develop a vocabulary to talk with patients and families about spirituality in such a way as to enhance the quality of the care we provide them? How can we best work collaboratively with ministers, counselors, and other spiritual professionals in caring for people across the full spectrum of their distress?

This book is written to allow physicians and patients to address important issues regarding the quality and meaning of all our lives. Twenty-first-century healthcare will inevitably have to face complex issues and challenges about care at the end of life, care of chronic and disabling illness, and complex ethical and moral dilemmas. At present, our ability to do these things can best be described as rudimentary. We hope that this book will be useful to practicing healthcare professionals. For them, it should provide a useful framework to improve their understanding of patients and their ability to communicate more intimately with them and their families. The book should also be useful for ministers and other spiritual professionals by providing a broader context for working with physicians and other healthcare workers. Finally, we hope this book can provide a much-needed foundation for medical students, nursing students, and seminary students, for anyone learning about the caring professions. It is our contention that the future of healthcare will be built on interdisciplinary teams of professionals that are equipped to address the full range of human suffering and triumph experienced by those in need. It is with this future in mind that we offer this text.

Stephen P Kliewer
John Saultz
September 2005

About the authors

Stephen P Kliewer D.Min. is the Executive Director of Wallowa Valley Center for Wellness, a nonprofit agency that provides mental health, alcohol and drug, and developmental disability programs for a small rural county in the State of Oregon (USA). Dr Kliewer is also an Assistant Professor in the Department of Family Medicine at Oregon Health & Science University (OHSU). At OHSU Dr Kliewer has been involved in curriculum development, program development and teaching. His areas of focus have been patient and physician communication, spirituality and medicine, mental health and primary care integration, and rural issues. To date he has participated in the writing of 49 funded grants and was directly involved in the implementation of 40 of those grants. Some highlights of his activities include the development and implementation of a cross-cultural medicine initiative and the development of a curriculum for predoctoral students and residents on the integration of healthcare and spirituality. Dr Kliewer was also the Project Coordinator for a primary care development project in Baku, Azerbaijan, funded through the American International Health Alliance (Washington, DC).

Dr Kliewer received a BA from Whitman College in Walla Walla, Washington, graduating with a double major in philosophy and English literature. He went on to receive a Masters in Divinity from Princeton Theological Seminary in Princeton, New Jersey and a Doctorate of Ministry from San Francisco Theological Seminary in San Anselmo, California. He is currently working on a Masters in Mental Health Counseling. For 14 years he was a pastor in the Presbyterian Church, USA serving three churches. In 1990 he joined NW Medical Teams International, a medical nonprofit agency involved in both disaster relief and medical development projects. He worked for NWMTI for four years and was involved in relief and development projects worldwide. His main area of focus was the development of health initiatives in rural Mexico. In 1994 he joined Oregon Health & Science University and in 2003 became the Director at Wallowa Valley Center for Wellness.

Dr Kliewer has published one book, *Creative Use of Diversity in the Local Church* (The Alban Institute, Washington, DC, 1987), and recently authored an article on medicine and healthcare published in the *Journal of Family Practice* (August 2004).

John W Saultz MD is Professor and Chairman, Department of Family Medicine at Oregon Health & Science University. Dr Saultz received his BS and MD degrees from Ohio State University. He completed his residency in family practice at Dwight David Eisenhower Army Medical Center, and a faculty development fellowship at the University of North Carolina at Chapel Hill.

From 1986 to 1994 Dr Saultz was the family practice residency director at Oregon Health & Science University. He is currently Chair of Family Medicine, Assistant Dean for Primary Care of the School of Medicine, and Director of the Oregon statewide Area Health Education Centers (AHEC) Program. In 2003–04, Dr Saultz was named a Bishop/American Council on Education Fellow.

Dr Saultz is a Diplomate of the American Board of Family Practice, a Fellow of the American Academy of Family Physicians, and a member of the Society of Teachers of Family Medicine.

Dr Saultz was the 1993–94 President of the Association of Family Practice Residency Directors and he was the 1996–97 President of the Oregon Academy of Family Physicians. Dr Saultz has served on the Residency Review Committee for Family Practice from 1999–2005 and on the Accreditation Council for Graduate Medical Education from 1992–98.

Dr Saultz is the author of *The Textbook of Family Medicine: defining and examining the discipline.* His current research interests include continuity of care in the doctor–patient relationship, medical decision making, and the future of family medicine.

CHAPTER 1

Healing, cure, and the whole person

> I cannot go to cure the body of my patient, but I
> forget my profession, and call unto God for his soul.
>
> Thomas Browne, *Religio Medici*

She had been his patient for over 20 years. An elderly woman with severe arthritis, she was the piano teacher for generations of children in her small rural community. She served as the accompanist for various school choirs and had been, for as long as anyone could remember, the pianist and organist for her church. Now her condition had worsened to the point that her deformed hands no longer allowed her to play her instrument. During a routine visit her physician noted the progression of her disease and empathized with her. 'I know that the pain associated with your conditions is really a problem. I want you to know that I will do everything I can to make you comfortable.' Her response had a profound impact on her dedicated and sensitive physician. 'Doctor, you don't understand. It is not the pain that is a problem. The problem is that I no longer know who I am.'

This woman had no family. She had no spouse, no children, no grandchildren. Outside of her work as a teacher and performer, she had no active involvement in the community. If she was not 'the piano teacher,' the 'school accompanist,' the 'church organist,' who was she? How was she to be defined? Clearly her disease involved more than the mere presence of a physical ailment. The complexity of her condition involved the totality of who she was as a human being.

As we explore what it means to provide effective healthcare to the whole person, one of the first issues we must address is the nature of personhood. What are the facets of a human being, and how do these facets and complexities impact how we practice healthcare? The modern clinical model, as it emerged from the Enlightenment and the consequent development of the scientific method, diminished the importance of the whole person and narrowed the focus of medicine to an almost one-dimensional plane. In the book *Patient-Centered Care*, Ian McWhinney relates the clinical method as described by Laennec, a French clinician writing in the early 1800s. Laennec, who is known as the discoverer of auscultation and inventor of the stethoscope, did an exhaustive 12-year study of chest-related disease. He attributed his discoveries to proper observation and described his methodology as follows (from *De l'auscultation mediate*):[1]

> The constant goal of my studies and research has been the solution of the following three problems:
> 1 To describe disease in the cadaver according to the altered states of the organs.

2 To recognize in the living body definite physical signs, as much as possible independent of the symptoms ...

3 To fight the disease by means which experience has shown to be effective; ...to place, through the process of diagnosis, internal organic lesions on the same basis as surgical disease.

By the late 1800s this method of strict observation and repeated testing had evolved into the modern clinical method for examining disease, and it has essentially defined medicine as we understand it today.

What is critical for this discussion is the focus on the physical aspect of disease created by this methodology. Emerging from this new investigative model was an understanding of disease as an essentially independent entity located in a host body. Over time, the medical community seems to have anthropomorphized diseases, endowing them with an essentially personal and independent existence. A functional disassociation between the disease and the person in whose body it resides has occurred. The mental, emotional, social, and spiritual aspects of the person are seen as secondary to the physical pathology. It is not unusual, in a hospital hallway, to hear two clinicians talking about 'the cancer' in room 401, or 'the cirrhosis' in room 503. The person with the disease fades into the background, and the importance of the patient's history, relationships, values, beliefs, fears, hopes, and dreams are lost.

But can a model of healing that focuses on the physical aspects of disease while neglecting the other facets of personhood be effective? Perhaps – if the absence of disease is the solitary goal of healthcare. But what if we have broader goals? In his book *Integrating Spirituality Into Treatment*, psychiatrist William Miller makes the following suggestion.

> If health is more than the absence of disease, and broader than the single dimension of suffering, then a healer's task is larger than the detection and eradication of a specific disease state. It has to do with quality of life, with the richness that is invoked when we truly ask and answer the question 'how are you?'[2]

Miller goes on to assert that health involves three domains. True health he suggests requires not only (1) the absence of suffering, but also (2) the presence of an ability to function and (3) what he calls 'coherence,' or what many call inner peace. Coherence is the ability to make sense of life and its events, to endow them with meaning. To be well one must weave coherence into the process of healing; one must identify the meaning one has conferred on the disease, and from that base of meaning find the capacity to function. Thus to be a healer means not only to address the physical aspect of the condition, relieving suffering and enhancing or restoring the physical capacity to function, but also to address the issue of coherence and enhance the emotional, spiritual, mental capacity to function. Being a healer means helping patients understand the meaning of their disease. Helping them place the disease in the context of their values and beliefs.

Brown, Weston and Steward capture the same concept when they insist that there is 'a distinction between two concepts of ill health: disease and illness... *Disease*, on the one hand, is an abstraction, the 'thing' that is wrong with the body-as-machine. *Illness*, on the other hand, is the patient's personal experience of sickness – the thoughts feelings and altered behaviors of someone who feels sick

... A particular disease is what everyone with that disease has in common, but the illness experience of each person is unique.'[3] Focusing on these two concepts these authors also approach wellness from a multifaceted perspective. Wellness requires dealing with the *disease* present in the body, the traditional task of medicine. But it also requires working with patients to address other aspects of their *illness*, their ideas and feelings, their expectations regarding treatment and outcomes, and their ability to function.[4] When the person is struggling with these other aspects they are experiencing what might be called 'dis-ease.' Dis-ease is a lack of peace or comfort centered in the non-physical aspects of the person. Dis-ease relates to the emotional, spiritual, and relational. What is common to both of these models is a broadened concept of personhood.

Personhood in faith systems

Since the beginning of recorded history there has been a sense that the physical body does not define a person. Both Jewish and Christian thought, for example, have always presented an image of the self as being multifaceted. The most common Judeo-Christian image of the self involves a dichotomy, involving both a body (*soma* in Greek, *basar* in Hebrew) and a soul (*psyche* in Greek, *nephesh* in Hebrew). In the Hebrew the word *basar* means, literally, 'flesh,' and by extension refers to the human body, with a focus on created life as opposed to divine life. It is often used along with the word *esem*, or bone, to convey unmistakably the idea of the physical body (flesh and bone). The word 'body' refers, importantly, to only the external form of the person. It is only one of the facets of the person, the other being the *nephesh* or soul (in a few cases the word *leb*, or heart, is used instead). According to John Oswalt, in the *Theological Wordbook of the Old Testament*, 'it would be inappropriate to think that the Hebrews conceived of a living soul inhabiting an otherwise dead body. Rather they saw the human reality as permeating all the components with the totality being the person.'[5] Often, in the Torah, the words 'soul' and 'body' are used together, illustrating the essential unity of the person. This is most evident in the Psalms:

> 'My soul longs, yea longs for the courts of the Lord, my heart and my
> flesh cry out for the living God.'
> Psalm 84:2

It must be noted however, that although the Jewish scriptures suggest a critical unity between body and soul, there are also hints of what is often called 'anthropological dualism.' The very use of dual terms for the self seems to indicate a number of unique components, each with their own reality. Although the soul and body have an essential unity and together are used to describe the corruptible self, there is also a degree of separation. 'The body may be seen at a certain remove. One may abandon it to pain or death, for the true I is the soul or reason which survives death.'[6]

A similar dichotomy is found in the writings of the New Testament. There the *soma* is the organic or corporeal body and is that which experiences sickness and healing (Mark 5:29) or needs food and clothing (James 2:16). However, as in Hebrew thinking, the body and the soul are not easily distinguished in the New Testament. Indeed, early Christian writers such as Paul reflect an even more profound connection between these two facets of the individual. Perhaps the best illustration of this essential unity is in the fact that the future life (life after death or life after the apocalypse), initiated by the resurrection, is a bodily one. According to Paul a person, when he or she is reunited with God, will be united 'even to the point of his corporeality.'[7]

The soul, in the New Testament, is the 'principle of all life, physical, intellectual, moral, religious.'[8] It has continued existence after the death of the body because God wills that the living principle of the human continue. The New Testament usage of the word *psyche* flows out of the common Greek usage of the word by philosophers such as Plato. In Greek thought the word 'psyche' was used to describe the life principle, or vital principle. The psyche was the organ of thought and judgment and often was seen as the immortal part of the person (Plato, *Timaeus 30B*).

There is a third word which must be included in any exploration of the concept of person in the Judeo-Christian tradition. That word is 'Spirit' (*pneuma* in the Greek and *ruah* in the Hebrew). There are some who would insist that the Spirit comprises a third additional facet of the total person. For these thinkers the soul is still defined as the principle of life, and includes understanding, emotion, and sensibility. But it is united with the corporeal in such a manner that it, along with the body, ceases to exist at death. The spirit, which literally means 'wind' or 'breath,' is, for this group, 'the mind, the principle of man's rational and immortal life, the possessor of reason, will, and conscience.'[9] At death the spirit returns to God who gave it.

If we were to query modern Christians about their concept of the person, and specifically their view regarding life after death, we would find this functional trichotomy widespread. Paul, and probably most early Christians, believed in the imminent return of Christ and a general corporeal resurrection of the dead. But as the years turned into decades, and the decades into centuries, the idea of an eventual physical resurrection was not enough for many believers. They wanted a sense that when a person died the transition to new, eternal life was more immediate. The concept of one's spirit being reunited with God in 'heaven' became a common solution among believers in general. It should be noted that many who hold to the concept of a dichotomy come up with the same solution to the problem of a delayed resurrection of the dead. For them the soul leaves the body and returns to God, a solution that, while emotionally satisfying, ignores the intrinsic unity of the body and soul portrayed in the New Testament.

For most Christians, however, the word 'Spirit' is used to describe not a third facet of personhood, but the dynamic presence of God in the person of the Holy Spirit. This Spirit comes into the person who is in relationship with God and possesses and influences that person, body and soul, so that the person lives in union with God and has a life that reflects God's presence. Their actions, indeed their very character, are transformed by the wind or breath of God.

In talking about the main thrust of Judeo-Christian thought, therefore, it is best to think primarily in terms of the classic dichotomy of body and soul. Soul, however, should be seen as complex in nature, being the locus of understanding or rational values and emotion. But even if affirming the dichotomy, we should not ignore the Spirit. For Christians the person, body and soul, is meant to be a person in relationship with the divine, connected to that power by the Spirit, which dwells within and becomes, essentially, a part of the person. The spiritual dimension, although not a component of the person itself, transforms the body/soul complex in which it dwells. Thus in a real sense it is appropriate to talk about the person as physical, soulful, and spiritual and insist that any approach to healing must include all of these elements.

The Sufi teacher Hazrat Inayat Khan presents a similar model of personhood in his book *The Inner Life*. According to this Muslim leader the purpose of life is 'to not only live in the body, but to live in the heart, to live in the soul.'[10] To see the self merely as a body is to be severely limited and to 'not know that another part of his being exists, which is much higher, more wonderful, more living, and more exalted.'[11] For Khan, in parallel with Judeo-Christian thought, to live as a multi-dimensional being is possible only as one connects with God. Indeed, the 'first and principle thing in the inner life is to establish a relationship with God, making God the object which we relate to ... '[12] So the person is multifaceted and is empowered by an inner connection to the divine.

The Buddhist concept of the person represents a significant departure from the family of faiths represented by the Judaism, Christianity, and Islam. It is best understood if one focuses on some concepts central to Buddhism. One of the most critical of these concepts is that of Nirvana. According to Huston Smith, a noted scholar of comparative religion, the word means to 'blow out' or 'to extinguish.'[13] It may be best to place the concept of Nirvana in the context of the Four Noble Truths, which explain the reality of life. The First Noble Truth is that life is *dukkha*, or suffering. It is not that life is nothing but suffering, as in Buddhism it is possible to experience joy in life. It is more that joy is superficial, and that at some level pain seeps into all finite existence. This pain exists because life is dislocated. The word *dukkha* is used in Pali to refer to an axle, which is off-center with respect to its wheel. Because things are 'off-center' or out of balance there is a resultant friction. Life 'rubs' and is full of conflict, barriers, and pain. Buddha in his teachings cited six occasions when life's dislocation is most evident: The trauma of birth, the pathology of sickness, the morbidity of decrepitude, the phobia of death, one's slavery to what one abhors, and one's separation from what one loves. So human life, in its normal condition, is out of balance, estranged, so to speak, from the truth, and this estrangement must be overcome if the pathologies of life are to be addressed and authentic happiness is to be achieved.

The Second Noble Truth points to the cause of this estrangement. We are out of balance, and thus in friction because of *tanha*, or the desire to seek fulfillment through the self. One writer calls *tanha* 'the desire for self at the expense, if necessary, of all other forms of life.'[14] The ego, as normally understood and nurtured by humans, is a barrier to fulfillment. The more we seek to satisfy the ego or self, the more it hinders our understanding of others as fellow participants of the same reality, and the more it hinders our ability to act for the benefit of the whole. The result is pain.

The Third Noble Truth focuses on the cure for humanity's pain. If we would get rid of the dislocation or imbalance that causes pain, we must get rid of the self-centeredness that causes it. We must move from the narrow imprisoning focus on the self and focus on the universal. The Fourth Noble Truth reveals that *tanha* can be overcome by following the Eightfold Path, which might be seen as spiritual principles, disciplines, or steps.

Nirvana, which is the state of balance that all seek, is thus not so much the extinguishing of the self, but elimination of the distinction between the individual self and the universal. It is not obliteration or self-annihilation, but, in a powerful sense, self-realization. It is coming into balance, and being what one was created to be, a person in a seamless, giving relationship with the whole. This is a difficult concept to comprehend. Buddha himself insisted that Nirvana was 'incomprehensible, indescribable, inconceivable, unutterable,' for if we eliminate every component of the self we understand, how can we speak of what is left?[15] Nirvana is not God, and many would argue that there is no concept of God in Buddhism. However, it might be safe to say that Nirvana is the realm of the Spiritual. So the self is best understood not in terms of the individual, but in terms of the universal, the wholeness that is the spiritual, an idea that is revolutionary for our perception of the goal of healthcare.

One of the more interesting aspects of Buddhist thought regarding the self is that people do not have a soul (or *atman*). There is no spiritual substance which can be seen separately from the physical self (no dualism) and retain its separateness beyond death. This denial of spiritual substance is part of a wider denial of substance. In Buddhism both the idea of permanence and matter are viewed with suspicion. For Buddha 'the mind was far more basic in man and nature than matter' and he 'challenged the implications of permanence contained in the idea of substance.'[16] Buddha thus viewed the body as rather ephemeral, a pile of elements no more permanently or concretely bound together than the grains of a sand pile.

So what are we left with? If the body is impermanent, and the soul is without substance, what is the essence of a person? Perhaps a clue can be found in discussions around life after death, or continuance. In Buddhism it is probably not correct to say either that a person 'lives on,' or that a person 'ceases to exist.' The first comment suggests a continuance of the individual that is not consistent with Buddha's thought. The second comment suggests total extinction, which is also inconsistent with what Buddha believed. Smith suggests a path somewhere between those two poles. 'The ultimate destiny of the human spirit is a condition in which all identification with the historical experience of the finite self will disappear while experience itself not only remains but is heightened beyond anticipation.'[17] There is a self or spirit which is part of a greater whole. It finds freedom and joy as it participates in that whole, and pain as it seeks distinction or separation. It finds peace as it moves from its ties to the temporal world, and a temporal body.

So with Buddhism, as with the Western faiths, there is a clear need to move beyond the body in the definition of the self, and a need to take the spiritual seriously in any attempt to bring healing into the presence of disease.

Philosophical and psychological definitions of personhood

During the last century a number of thinkers attempted to define personhood. One of those people was Paul Tournier, a physician from Switzerland, who presents at the beginning of his book *The Whole Person in a Broken World* what he considers the prevailing image of the person in the world of medicine.

> What, then, is the person? ...Everybody knows what direction medical science has pursued for a hundred years now in order to answer that question. It has pursued the direction of materialism. And from that point

of view man is compared with a machine, or more precisely, with an assemblage of machines ... man is a complex ensemble of different machines – digestive system, respiratory, nervous, urinary systems, etc. ...[18]

The direction of medical science has, Tournier admits, created great advances in knowledge, but in its reduction of people to the merely physical and medicine to physical pathology, it has become limited and unbalanced. Tournier points to Freud, who he insists, 'broke the line of the development of organic pathological medicine and rediscovered the importance of the psychic,'[19] showing that there are problems that are not caused by a lesion, but by an idea (again we move toward the concept of dis-ease). According to Tournier, if it is true that there are both organic diseases and non-organic 'functional' diseases based on such things as imagination, then medicine must look beyond the body to a broader definition of the person. He echoes here the thoughts of Alexis Carrel, who insists that we cannot perceive the material, mental, and spiritual aspects of the human as different things. 'Neither the soul nor the body can be investigated separately. We observe merely a complex being whose activities have been arbitrarily divided into physiological and mental.'[20] Tournier ultimately concludes that any adequate conception of the person must be one that includes the body, psychological functions, and something more, what most would call the soul or spirit. Only this kind of transformed vision of the person will allow us to truly bring healing into people's lives.

One author who provides such a conception is Dr Jean de Rougemont. According to de Rougemont human life manifests itself through five different phenomena:[21]

1   bodily, physical phenomena
2   psychic phenomena: the play of imagination, the interior sense
3   mental phenomena: abstract thinking, judgment, and reasoning
4   unconscious phenomena
5   spiritual phenomena.

These five phenomena make up four levels of being, the physical, psychic, mental, and spiritual. The unconscious phenomena do not constitute a level of being, but are instead incorporated into all levels except the physical. Psychic, mental, and spiritual phenomena can be either conscious or unconscious. It is important to note that although de Rougemont differentiates between these various levels and types of phenomena, he believes in a critical unity similar to the unity between body and soul seen in the religious models of personhood. 'We are "men" through our body, our psyche, our mind, our unconscious, and our spirit... there are no sharp boundaries.'

Alex Stocker developed a similar model in his book *The Confusion of Modern Man*. Stocker uses a triangle to define the various components of the person. At the pinnacle is the heart (A), which as he defines it, is very similar to the Biblical concept of spirit. The middle section represents the mental or intellectual aspect of the person (B), and the base of foundation of the pyramid is the body (C), or the physical.

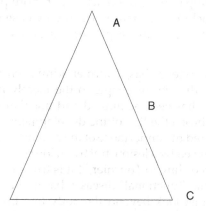

Figure 1.1

Tournier, who followed them, refers to both de Rougemont and Stocker in his deliberations. However, although he clearly appreciates the models they have developed, he feels that both their models are insufficient to explain the complexity of the person, especially with respect to the presence of the spirit. The spirit, he notes, which is present at the apex of Stocker's model, and as the final level of de Rougemont's, is clearly different from the other components of the self. 'One can make body, psyche, and the mind the object of experiment. The spirit, however, is inaccessible to science; it can be perceived only intuitively, introspectively, or better, through grace.'[22]

Therefore Tournier suggests yet another model of the person, one which incorporates the spirit in a more inclusive and intimate manner. For him the spirit essentially permeates the entire self, body (A), as well as the psyche (B) and mind (C). It is the spirit that brings life to all of them. The spirit is the point of intersection between all the aspects of the person, and perhaps also the point of intersection between the person and the sacred.

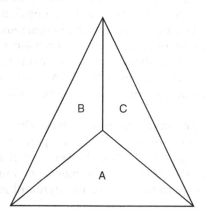

Figure 1.2

The spirit, as a point of intersection, is essentially without dimension, and thus is not accessible except through the other aspects of the person. But it can be expressed through the body (through actions), through the psyche (through feelings or perhaps art), and through the mind (through the world of ideas – perhaps theology).

This model shows more clearly than the others we have explored why the modern clinical method has had such a difficult time incorporating the spiritual aspect of the person. By adopting the scientific method, medicine became totally dependent upon objective investigation of things that can be seen and measured. Therefore it is condemned to understanding only those aspects of the person that encompass the 'exterior' components, the body, psyche, and mind. Since it cannot directly access the spiritual aspect of the person, it ignores this critical component that defines the person we see, touch, and hear. In short, according to Tournier's model of the person, medicine misses that which ultimately defines the person.

It seems important to include at least one model of the person emerging from the world of psychotherapy. Virginia Satir, in her book *Peoplemaking*, talks about the various aspects of personhood in a very functional manner. She believes there are four aspects that demand attention:[23]

- the feelings and ideas one has about himself, *self-worth*
- the ways people work to make meaning with one another, *communication*
- the *rules* people use for how they should feel and act, which eventually develop into the family system
- the way people relate to other people and institutions outside the family, or the *link to society*.

These four aspects relate both to how a person functions internally (emotionally) and how they function within their family and within society (socially). These aspects also relate to the rules or values by which a person lives, to the way they see life, respond to life events, and establish meaning. So, in essence, they also relate to the existential or spiritual.

Satir's model, although clearly not developed from any sort of religious perspective, is very consistent with the models we explored earlier. Again we see both the complexity and essential unity of the person. She does not, since she is developing a psychological model, address the issue of the body, but does create added dimension to the non-physical aspects of personhood by focusing on the social or interpersonal.

In the religious models, as well as those of Tournier, Stocker, and de Rougemont, the vertical relationship between the person and something, someone beyond the self are explicit. Indeed, in many of these models it is this vertical relationship that defines the person. This is especially clear in Tournier's model, with its spiritual axis. Satir's model introduces the horizontal relationship between the person and other people and addresses this relationship as an essential part of the model. While in many of the other models the person cannot be defined without taking into account the connection to that which is greater, or beyond the self, however defined, in Satir the person cannot be defined without taking into account the connection between that person and other people. Indeed one of her categories relates to the person's 'inner' relationships, the psyche, mind, and spirit, while three of her categories relate to the person's outer relationships. These rules and values define the way the person interacts with others, the methods by which they communicate, and the linkages that are created.

The person defined

There are then, a variety of ways in which one can define personhood. It seems that at the very least we must include two aspects, body and soul (or spirit). However, in order to better capture the complexity of human nature it is better to include four basic components.

- First there is the body, the physical aspect of the person and the focus of disease-centered medicine.
- Second there is what we might call the soul, the realm of the 'inner person.' This might include one's thoughts, feelings, perhaps that part of our self that is impacted and imprinted by our personal histories.
- Third there is the social self. The self as it functions within the context of a shared humanity. The self in relationship with others, including significant others, families, peers, and co-workers. This aspect of the self relates to our horizontal relationships.
- Finally there is the spiritual self, the self as it relates to something greater than itself, however that might be defined.

It must be noted that separating these four aspects into distinct factors is artificial. As has been noted by almost all of the thinkers we have explored, there is an essential unity of personhood, a significant linkage between all of the facets of personhood, with each of them connecting to and impacting the others. So it is that if something happens to us physically, it affects us socially, spiritually, and relationally. This is why it makes sense to talk about the 'meaning' of a disease for the patient. How do they connect the dots? What does their cancer mean to them on a spiritual level? Do they see it as a curse, some sort of punishment, as something that is meant to test their faith, or as a chance event that their connection to the sacred will enable them to manage? What is the impact on their inner self? Does it make them bitter and cynical or does it create a new capacity for empathy? How does it impact their significant relationships? Is it a barrier to intimacy, or something that creates a new intimacy?

To take any one facet of the individual and focus on it to the exclusion of the others is to err. For the physician to ask that the patient leave their spiritual/social/inner self at the door and bring in only the physical self is inappropriate, just as it would be inappropriate for a minister to treat the spirit or soul, but ignore the social or physical aspects of the self. To preach 'salvation' to a person who is hungry is just as improper as treating a person for physical pain, but ignoring the presence of spiritual or emotional suffering.

Let us look at these four facets of self as they present in one person. Developing this kind of a portrait helps us to see how these various facets unfold in the therapeutic relationship between a patient and a provider. Let us begin with the purely physiological facet of the patient.

Harvey is a 62-year-old African American man who has been hospitalized due to worsening of his chronic lung condition. He developed worsening shortness of breath about four years ago. As the symptom worsened, he became unable to walk up the stairs to his apartment and could not make the trip downstairs to his mailbox each day. Harvey consulted his physician who discovered an abnormality in his chest x-ray and referred him to a lung specialist. After a series of tests, a diagnosis of interstitial pulmonary fibrosis was made. The doctors explained to Harvey that this condition was caused by a gradual process in which the lungs become infiltrated with fibrous tissue causing them to become stiff and leathery. He was told that this condition is usually progressive and that he would not get better. Although there are medications to slow the disease process, only a lung transplant had any chance of restoring him to a functional life. Prior to his hospitalization, a visiting nurse came to his home every day to help him with his daily care needs. He depends on oxygen around the clock to avoid feeling short of breath when simply sitting in a chair.

So far we have defined our patient in terms of the physical self, and see him only from the perspective of the disease that is attacking his body. But clearly Harvey is more than a physical body, he is a person.

Harvey is a retired mail carrier who was married, but is now divorced and living alone. He is also a father, with two adult daughters who live in other states. He corresponds infrequently with one of these daughters and is completely estranged from the other. Harvey is a man with few friends, but prior to his illness he regularly visited a community senior citizens' center and enjoyed playing cards.

Now Harvey is beginning to emerge as a real person, with his social or relational self slowly gaining definition. In this case we have a person whose relational facet is marked by failure and isolation.

Since learning of his diagnosis, he has felt angry and despondent, but he hasn't talked with anyone about these feelings. Within the past week, Harvey was told that he probably would not qualify for a lung transplant due to his lack of social support and his other medical problems. He tearfully admits to being afraid and is desperate for any hope of treatment for his condition.

Now we are in the realm of the inner person, the soul. Harvey has revealed something of his inner self and we begin to see his feelings regarding his disease and how he is allowing that disease to define his life. We have a glimpse at a deeper level of how this person thinks and feels, how he responds to the challenges life presents. We begin to understand that there is a condition here that goes beyond the interstitial pulmonary fibrosis. This is a person profoundly afflicted at the level of the heart, a man who is suffering in the realm of the soul. But what about the realm of the spiritual?

Harvey is not a person who displays an overt spirituality. He does not attend church, and has not shared any sort of spiritual history. Yet spiritual issues are clearly present. This is a person who is living on what might be called the dark side of spirituality. He is full of fear, hopelessness, and isolation. He not only has few relational resources to draw upon, but also few spiritual resources. He has no clear sense of connection with the divine, no sense of comfort or hope, but instead, a profound dread of the future and death. Thus his spirituality is not likely to be of much help in coping with his illness.

Because of where he is spiritually, his physical condition is likely to be overwhelming, and the possibility that he will find healing in the midst of his illness (both his disease and his dis-ease), that he will be able to tap into his spirituality and find blessing in the midst of disease, is low. Since the research shows that a positive spirituality can be very effective in helping people cope with chronic or terminal disease,[24] Harvey might well benefit if his spirituality could be nurtured and he could find empowerment at that level.

Questions for reflection

- If you were to define 'the self' how would you do it? (What are the components of the self from your perspective?)
- What aspect of your self do you consider most important? Which aspect has the most influence on how you live life?

The realm of the spiritual

Now that a concept of the person has been developed that is multifaceted and includes the realm of the spiritual, it is time to move forward and define spirituality more clearly. In order to define the rather nebulous concept of spirituality we must first differentiate it from the concept of religion. What is religion? According to those exploring the relationship of medicine and spirituality, religion has certain unique characteristics.

- Religious factors are focused heavily on prescribed beliefs, rituals, and practices, as well as social institutional features.[25]
- Being religious involves undertaking the search for the sacred (for God, meaning, purpose, truth, fulfillment) using specific means or methods (such as rituals or behaviors) within an identifiable group of people.[26]
- Religion is an organized social entity.[27]
- Religion is a specific system of belief, worship, conduct, etc., often involving a code of ethics and a philosophy.[28]

If we look at these brief descriptions, we see that religion is seen to be communal or social by nature. But it is not just communal. It is also 'organized.' People do not merely spend time together, they do so within an organized and defined context. There are specific agreed-upon rituals, formalized modes of worship. People not only gather, but when they gather their togetherness is based on a standardized set of beliefs and values. Religions usually have a designated corpus of writings deemed as core or sacred and various symbols that represent this sacred reality. The group also sets or establishes norms for behavior, not only within the community of faith, but also within daily life. In general, the community and the reality it represents have a certain degree of authority over the individual. In other words, the individual is subservient to the corporate. Perhaps the most positive way to view religion is to see it as a means rather than as an end. It is a way to develop, to pursue spiritual growth. People participate in a religion, adhering to its beliefs, values, and practices, in order to find their place both in terms of the sacred and the worldly. It is a way to search for closeness with the sacred, and a way to understand one's purpose in the world or universe. As many people will be quick to note, participation in a religion does not guarantee that a person is spiritual. Many people participate in religion out of habit, or because of cultural norms. Some may participate in religion for very non-spiritual reasons, such as profit, political or social advancement, even relational peace.

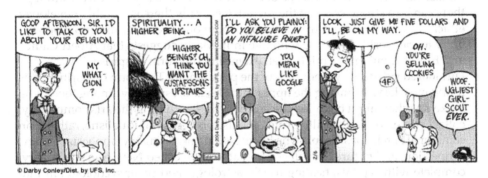

© Darby Conley/Dist. by UFS, Inc.

Figure 1.3

Get Fuzzy © Darby Conley. Distributed by United Feature Syndicate, Inc.

But in spite of the fact that there are those who practice religion out of very un-spiritual motives, many people are both religious and spiritual.

So what is spirituality? This concept is not an easy one to define and there have been many attempts to explain spirituality in meaningful terms. Definitions that have emerged from the medical literature are as follows.

- Spirituality is better understood as a multidimensional space in which every individual can be located.[29]
- Spiritual factors ... are concerned more with individual subjective experiences, sometimes shared with others.[30]
- Spirituality is a search for what is sacred or holy in life, coupled with some kind of transcendent (beyond self) relationship with God or a higher power or universal energy.[31]
- Spirituality connotes an individual's private search for meaning and connection, particularly his or her relationship with God.[32]

These definitions share some common elements. In each case, spirituality is seen as private or individualistic, rather than communal or social. Thus, while spirituality may be experienced communally, it is seen as an inherently personal or subjective experience. Second, spirituality is generally seen as experiential in nature. It has less to do with doctrines, ideas, or even rituals, and more to do with inner feelings, movement, or impact within the world of emotions, the realm of the heart. It is not that spirituality does not involve practices or rituals, but these activities tend to be more individualistic rather than organized or formal, and are geared at stimulating inner movement or growth.

Martin E Marty, a Protestant theologian and church historian, insists that spirituality is generally 'moored' or connected, however loosely, to some sort of religious tradition. Within the United States he has identified five types of spirituality, each unique due to the religious tradition to which it is moored most tightly.[33]

- **Humanistic spirituality** (in the US about 7% of the population): This type of spirituality focuses on the human spirit. People espousing this kind of spirituality believe that the individual can, through the nurturing of the spiritual facet, grow and develop, essentially becoming self-transcendent. There is generally no transcendent reference, no sense of a deity or even of a higher power, although there can be a strong sense of the sacred. Generally there is a highly developed ethical system involving strong feelings about one's relationship and responsibility to the world and those who live in it. Marty suggests that Albert Camus and Ernest Hemingway might well exemplify this form of spirituality.
- **Unmoored spirituality** (about 7% of the population): This form of spirituality is found most heavily among the upper middle class, especially among those who make up what might be called the cultural elite, including the arts community, college professors, and health professionals. It is very individualistic, rather than communal or religious. People who have this kind of spirituality emphasize energy, connection, and nature. Devotees of what is often called New Age spirituality, complete with crystals, healing touch, astrology, and parapsychology, fit into this form of spirituality, as do those who pursue their spirituality through books, taking bits and pieces from many faith systems and creating a hybrid spirituality. Some within this group maintain that they connect most effectively with the divine through nature. According to Marty this is the type of spirituality exemplified by Shirley MacLaine.
- **Moored spirituality – Eastern Type** (<3% of the population): A growing number of people in the United States, and a large number of people worldwide, fit into what Marty calls 'Eastern Type' spirituality. This group would include Buddhists, Taoists, Shintoists, and Hindus, all faith systems that espouse connection to a sacred core, to 'something' beyond or universal, but do not have a deity in the standard sense. The connection for those in this group would be to the sacredness of creation or to an indefinable universal other. This type of spirituality does involve practices, some of which are outer, or observable, but many of which might be classified as inner. This group would think more in terms of meditation than of prayer, more in terms of inner growth or inner peace than of divine intervention.
- **Moored spirituality – Western Type I** (about 25% of the US population): This group includes an eclectic collection of faith systems including evangelical and conservative Protestant Christians, Pentecostal Christians, Roman Catholics, Orthodox Christians (most varieties), Jews, and Muslims. In all of these groups there is a strong sense of the divine, of a deity to whom one is ultimately responsible. This deity is generally very authoritarian by nature and is in control of the world. Generally the deity is anthropomorphized and seen as a person who can be named, such as Yahweh, Allah, or Jesus. As a being who has been given form and substance, God is often assigned a role (often relating to an earthly or human role) such as king or father and can be visualized. A wonderful example of such visualization is Michelangelo's incredible painting of God passing the spark of life to Adam. People in this spiritual domain believe they can interact with the divine in a personal way, primarily through prayer. Some

from this group believe they regularly enter into what can actually be thought of as a dialogue with the divine. The sense of active interchange is stronger within some of the faith systems of this group than others. The critical distinction is that with this group, God is seen as not only being approachable, but as being responsive, intervening in people's lives. Many people from this domain believe that God is concerned with illness and intervenes, bringing cure and/or healing.

- **Moored spirituality – Western Type II** (about 60% of the US population): This group has some strong similarities to the Western Type I but consists of those who are on the more liberal side of the religious spectrum. This group includes most mainstream Protestant Churches, as well as some from the Roman Catholics, Orthodox Christians, Jews and Muslims. The fact that some of these groups are also included in Western Type I reflects the presence of diversity within those systems. This group has a similar view of God, although the 'image' of God in this system is likely to be less concrete and less defined. God is more like some sort of benevolent power, difficult to define and picture. It is not that God is less real to this group, merely that those within this type of spirituality tend to be less concrete in their visualization of God, and in their thinking. This group is also more likely to be tolerant and inclusive in terms of dogma. They will have less defined doctrines and fewer or more flexible rules of behavior. In short, this group has fewer issues which they see as 'black and white' and more that are perceived as 'gray', situational, or perhaps even subjective by nature. They believe that all of life is under 'God' and that we should live responsibly in terms of our own self, others, our communities (religious and otherwise), and even the natural world. This group also believes in prayer, but generally does not pray with the specificity of Western Type I. They will generally ask merely that 'God's will be done.' Those belonging to Western Type I sometimes see those in this group as being vague, unsure, or weak due to their reluctance to claim God's clear direction in daily life. In the uncertainty of the late twentieth and early twenty-first centuries, this type of spirituality, once dominant in America, has been fading while the more dogmatic, assertive, and definitive spirituality of Western Type I has been growing.

The distinctions outlined by Marty are helpful in understanding the broad range encompassed by the term 'spirituality.' Marty's typologies, because they encompass the breadth of human experience, suggest that all of us are spiritual beings, even those who are reluctant to adhere to any concept of the divine. There is a spiritual component (although it may not always be defined that way) even in those who totally reject the idea of a god or divine being, or reject the idea of a 'power greater than one's self.' Sometimes the spiritual component is well developed, and is both important and impactful. At other times the spiritual aspect of the person is buried or repressed, or merely undeveloped, and is not a visibly powerful part of the person's life. Sometimes it is clearly identified as 'spiritual' and at other times given another label (such as 'energy'). But it is our belief that the spiritual is there, in each of us, and that it is a part of the essential unity that makes up the individual person. It is also our belief that the spiritual is both a potential benefit and a potential barrier to the process of healing. It is something that both affects physical health and is affected by it. It is important therefore to respect spirituality and to understand the spiritual type one is working with. It is not critical that we use the spiritual types defined by Marty, as his typology is not exact or exhaustive. What is important is that we develop a paradigm for thinking about a person's spiritual mode so we can interface with them in an effective and sensitive manner.

We must also recognize that many people express their inner spirituality through the medium of religion. Religion, unlike spirituality, is centered on concrete observable components such as communities, sacred writings, images and icons, worship, and other outward observances. Religion provides content, with visible clues, and thus is often the point of focus when we think about or work in the realm of the spiritual. Most research that has been done on the integration of medicine and spirituality has really been research on religion not spirituality. It is informative that Koenig, McCullough, and Larson titled their exhaustive and academic look at the subject *The Handbook of Religion and Medicine*. The religious affiliation of a person can be an excellent clue about a person's spiritual mode, but is not an infallible indicator. As we saw in Marty's typology, some religious systems are contained in multiple types. In reality any effort to categorize a person's spirituality is fraught with difficulty. For example, a person can 'belong' to a faith system, due to cultural influence, family history, or other such factors, but in fact have a spiritual mode that is far different from that common to that system. A person can belong to a system but not truly be in touch with their spirituality at all. So one must be careful to avoid relying too heavily on religious affiliation while exploring another's spiritual perspective.

In general, when talking about spirituality, it is best to think in terms of a 'culture of one.' Each person's spirituality is different, shaped by a whole array of associated life factors including their personal history: their family, their culture, the religious community they grew up in (or the lack of such a religious background), their education, their friends, the books they have read. Spirituality is extremely personal, and is constantly evolving.

One author, in attempting to capture this dynamic, realistically states that we should focus on process not content. To focus on process is to focus on 'vague implicit bodily feelings in a special way so that they unfold and bring new explicit meanings that result in psychological relief or release.' On the other hand 'content involves symbolizations, or what the process is all about.'[34] To focus on the process allows the caregiver to focus on what is happening inside the spiritual facet of the individual, to look for growth or regression, for joy or agony. To focus on content means to focus on the outward signs and symbols, and thus on things that can be misunderstood. It is the process, this author insists, which is truly the spiritual, that which is common to all of us. The spiritual experience is 'a subtle, bodily feeling with vague meanings that brings new, clear meanings involving a transcendent growth process.'[35] Content is very specific to unique systems and cultures and often brings with it 'baggage' that leads to alienation or judgment.

As we work with people around those feelings, which can range from the subtle to the intense, and seek to help them establish fresh meaning and thus experience spiritual growth, we must move carefully and gently. Our role is that of a facilitator and our goal is nothing more (or less) than to help that person unwrap, reveal, perhaps discover their spirituality in our presence. Henri Nouwen, a Roman Catholic author, has a marvelous description, in his book *Reaching Out*, of what it means to take spirituality seriously, and work with a person in that sacred realm.[36]

> Hospitality means primarily the creation of a free space where the stranger can enter and become a friend instead of an enemy. Hospitality is not to change people, but to offer them space where change can take

place. It is not to bring men and women over to our side, but to offer freedom ... it is not an educated intimidation with good books, good stories, and good works, but the liberation of fearful hearts ... The paradox of hospitality is that it wants to create emptiness, not a fearful emptiness, but a friendly emptiness where strangers can enter and discover themselves as created free – free to sing their own song, speak their own languages, dance their own dances; free also to leave and follow their own vocations.[36]

Questions for reflection

- How do you define spirituality? Develop your own definition.
- How do you define religion?
- What is the relationship of spirituality and religion?
- What is your spiritual 'type'?

Health and healing

Before we move on from the task of developing functional definitions, it will be helpful to take a look at one more word, 'health.' Clearly the goal of healthcare should be to create or facilitate health. But what does that mean?

The concept of health is as complex as personhood. For many, it is impossible to think about health without thinking in terms of disease. In his book *The Tibetan Book of Healing*, Lopsang Rapgay notes, 'When we think about our health, we are actually accustomed to thinking in terms of disease... When we feel fine we rarely think about our health or what we need to do to maintain it.'[37] Normally, in other words, we define health as the absence of illness. This is not surprising, since, when it comes to our physical body, which is the most concrete and observable facet of the person, we tend to notice what is wrong more than appreciate what is right. We seem to expect to feel well, to have the 'machine' function properly, much in the same way we expect a car to simply 'run' when we turn the key. When everything works appropriately many of us simple don't pay attention, and thus don't have a well-defined sense of wellness. It may break through at times, when we accomplish something physically, or emerge from illness, or just have a burst of energy, but often wellness is taken for granted. It is when our biological 'machine' experiences a dysfunction that we take notice, and our sense is of being unwell or ill. What we must remember is that health has to do with both the presence and the absence of physical illness.

But we must also remember that illness and health are not simply about the physical. People also suffer from problems, such as pain, weakness, or exhaustion, which are more subjective than a fever or a tumor. People experience conditions that are more subjective and elusive still, such as suffering, loneliness, or a sense of loss. People also enjoy such experiences as joy, energy, and hope. Illness can be experienced not only in the realm of the physical, but also in the realms of the soul, the spiritual, or even the social. In these realms, as well as in the physical realm, it can be either positive or negative, the presence of health (or absence of illness), or the presence of illness (or absence of health).

Illness or health in one facet of life can carry over and affect other facets, or can remain relatively contained. A person can be ill with a physical disease such as cancer, but be healthy in all of the other facets of his or her personhood. Conversely a person can be ill socially or spiritually and yet be healthy physically (examples of non-transference). A person can be ill physically, and have that condition affect his spiritual life negatively, or have a spiritual or emotional condition that contributes to physical disease. This returns us to the essential unity of the person. We must remember that a problem in any one facet of personhood may, eventually, impact other facets negatively, while health in any facet may well impact the other facets positively. This is why the World Health Organization has defined health as 'a state of complete physical, mental and social well-being, and not the mere absence of disease or infirmity.' Rapgay similarly, insists that we must 'learn to recognize the role played by physical, psychological, emotional, social, spiritual and environmental factors in contributing to the overall quality of our lives.'[38]

One of the best definitions of health comes in the book from the American Psychological Association, *Integrating Spirituality into Treatment*. In an opening article, two of the contributors, Miller and Thoresen, suggest that health can be thought of has having three domains: suffering, function, and coherence.[39] *Suffering* defines the experience of the absence of health. Suffering may be experienced in many forms, such as physical pain, emotional pain, anxiety, depression, anger, or loneliness. *Function* defines one's functional ability. Can one function fully, or is one impaired? Again this is a complex dimension. Ability or impairment can be seen in every facet of the person. On the physical level we can look at such things as physical flexibility or strength, a functioning immune system, or a deficient one. On the social level we find people who can relate meaningfully to others, and those who can't. Emotionally one can be capable of naming, owning, and expressing deep emotions, or incapable and repressive. Spiritually one can be in touch with that which gives life meaning and purpose (functional), or out of touch (impaired). It is important to note that 'the impairment or loss of a particular function may be devastating to one person and irrelevant to another ...'[40] This is all very personal, and again it must be stressed that with each person we are dealing with a 'culture of one.'

The final aspect of health is *coherence*. Miller and Thoresen equate coherence with inner peace. It is a sense that life makes sense, there is meaning and purpose, and hope is a realistic option. Here we are dealing with a positive presence. Without the presence of this inner peace one can be physically well, free of disease, but not healthy. It has been suggested that we live in a time where a lack of coherence is rampant, at least in industrialized nations. In the past, most people in the world were needed to ensure survival. People were needed to provide food, clothing, heat, and transportation, all the necessities of life. A person's job might be difficult or unglamorous, but it was necessary if the family or the community were to survive. Now far fewer people are involved in such 'essential' activities. So many of the 'life support' functions in our society have become so mechanized that only a small percentage of the workforce is actually involved in performing them. Instead a large percentage of the workforce is involved in providing such products as recreation and entertainment, in tasks that are inherently less meaningful than survival tasks. It is far more difficult for people to find meaning, therefore, through their jobs. Meaning must be found in other ways, through relationships, volunteerism, or faith.

Also challenging coherence are the dynamics present in our world. DA Walrath, in his book *Frameworks*, suggests that there was a time when the world held life together.[41] Life was relatively confined and most aspects of life were integrated. Work, church, school, home, government, and leisure were connected in time and space, and generally included a specific group or community of people who shared many aspects of life in common. People not only lived next to their neighbors, but in many cases worshipped, worked, and played with them. People were interconnected. In some isolated rural areas this way of life still exists. But in much of the world this kind of life is gone. Life is faster, more complex, broader, and less reflective. The various components of life are often not related at all. It is common for neighbors to barely know each other, for people to work in communities other than those they live in, to never see co-workers outside of work, and for communities of worship to be totally separate from the daily world of the worshippers. Today's world no longer holds life together, it fragments it.

Another issue in today's world that challenges and disturbs a sense of coherence is change. There was a time when change happened so slowly it was hardly noticeable. There was change, but the changes were incremental, infrequent, and manageable. Now change is rapid and exponential. Ray Kurzweil is an inventor, an entrepreneur, an author, and a futurist. The creator of the first reading machine for the blind, speech recognition technology, and many other technologies that help envision the future, he is one of the most innovative creators of our time. It is his belief that we are experiencing an age of acceleration, a time when change not only happens, but also happens with increasing rapidity.

> In the first stage of human-directed technology, it took tens of thousands of years, which is what you would expect for the next stage via the wheel, or stone tools, and that kept accelerating, because when we had stone tools, we could use them to build the next stage. So a thousand years ago a paradigm shift only took a century, like the printing press. And now a paradigm shift, like the World Wide Web, is measured in only a few years' time.[42]

This accelerating change has a great impact on people. It creates uncertainty, confusion, and a loss of coherence. As Kurzweil notes, 'today there's an axiom that the only constant is change. But what people don't recognize is that the world itself has changed because the greater change is accelerating, so our whole concept of what it means to be human is going to be changing.'[43]

A final issue is the way in which world events confuse people and violate many of their expectations and values. The increase of technology is an excellent example. Back in the middle of the twentieth century, people, enamored with advances in technology and thrilled by voyages to the moon, came to expect that technology would eventually solve most of the problems faced by humanity. While technology has produced many benefits, it has not been the panacea it was hoped it would be. In fact technology has actually generated new challenges and threats. It was believed, for example, that medicine would find cures for most, if not all, diseases. Instead, medicine, while making progress, has not found the cure for all diseases. Indeed, new and frightening diseases such as AIDS and SARS have emerged, and we are even seeing drug-resistant versions of old diseases such as tuberculosis. It was believed we would find new ways to generate power that would be nearly inexhaustible. Our quest for effective new sources of power was sidetracked by Three Mile Island and Chernobyl. Our use of technology and our resource-hungry lifestyle have created major environmental issues that affect everything from our health to our weather.

Meanwhile many of things that rob people of wellness and happiness and hinder progress the most, things such as hatred, bigotry, and violence, continue unabated and are actually aided by our technology. We have become amazingly effective at killing one another. No wonder people struggle with the issues of meaning and purpose and find it difficult to establish the kind of coherence that Miller believes is a key to wellness. Not being able to make sense of the world contributes greatly to a sense of dis-ease.

Health then, can be seen as involving these three major modalities: suffering, function, and coherence. Using this definition we move from a definition of health that focuses on the body and physical disease to a more comprehensive, and hopefully useful, definition of health and healing.

> If health is more than the absence of disease, and broader than the single dimension of suffering, then a healer's task is larger than the detection and eradication of a specific disease state. It has to do with quality of life, with the richness that is invoked when we truly ask and answer the question, 'How are you?'[44]

From this perspective we see healing as much more than facilitating a physical cure. It must also involve a healing of the mind and emotions, the soul, a healing at the level of the spiritual and/or the social and relational. Cure has to do with the physical aspect of healing. Healing may involve cure, but is clearly much more. Healing may come, even when cure does not. A person may not find their physical disease eradicated, but they may find a sense of inner peace, or may find resolution in a fractured relationship, or they may rediscover a connection to the sacred in the midst of disease.

Back in 1980 Dr Paul Kliewer was a physician and surgeon in a small rural community in Oregon. Paul was an outstanding and well-loved doctor who lived an active and healthy lifestyle. He rarely drank alcohol and had never smoked in his life. He spent most of his free time outdoors, working in his yard, hunting, fishing, or hiking. He was extremely fit and had no apparent health problems. In the summer of 1980, Paul got a cold that would not go away and soon became progressively worse. Finally, when it was clear that there was at least a serious infection, his partner, also his son-in-law, convinced him to get some tests. The results were devastating. Paul had mesothelioma, an untreatable form of cancer commonly related to asbestos exposure.

The main tumor was located in the pleura, but by the time it was identified it had also spread to the lungs. It was clear that not much could be done from a medical perspective. His specialists recommended that he receive various kinds of treatment to shrink the tumor and provide some additional comfort, but offered no hope of cure. He decided that he would do nothing except control his pain. So much for the physical aspect of this illness.

Paul, the son of a Mennonite minister, was a man of faith. Since there was no Mennonite church in the small community he served, he had joined the Presbyterian Church and had been a regular attendee and an elder. Indeed, for his family, missing church was rarely an option. Even if he had spent the night delivering a baby, Sunday morning would find Paul in worship. The congregation became very used to the sight and sound of him asleep in the back pew, head back, snoring loudly.

When he received the news of his illness and the diagnosis that he might have as little as six months to live he decided to seek healing. He understood completely that healing in his case would probably not mean cure, and so approached the process in a unique way. He focused on all aspects of his personhood, and sought enrichment and healing in each sphere. Yes, he did take care of the physical side. Although he did not accept treatments such as radiation, he did take care of his body and sought to strengthen it in any manner possible. But his focus was clearly on other facets of his life. He reaffirmed his belief in God, and actively sought to nurture and build his sense of being connected to God: he started a small bible study group, read the Bible, read other religious writings, prayed, and participated in worship. He worked on the relational side of his life. All through his life he had been a very generous and kind person, but he had not been a person who easily showed or shared emotion. Now he consciously began developing that side of himself. He took extra time to visit with friends. He retired from practice and, with his fifth wheel trailer, made the rounds, visiting his brothers and sisters and his children. He traced his genealogy, and built relationships with many relatives he had never met. He worked hard at deepening his relationship with his brother, his wife, and his children. And he succeeded. In the process of deepening and nurturing his relationships with people and with God he built an inner life that could sustain him through the progression of his illness. Throughout his illness he was a stable person, with a clear sense of inner peace. In short, although Paul did not experience healing in the realm of the physical, he did in the realms of the emotional, social, and spiritual.

To look at his experience another way, although there was some physical suffering and even some emotional pain, overall Paul was able to move away from anxiety, depression, anger, and loneliness and toward community, hope, and joy. In the absence of overwhelming suffering, he enjoyed health. He stayed very functional. Even after his physical strength began to wane, he was able to stay active emotionally, relationally, and mentally. He continued, for example, to provide leadership for a study group. Again, we see the marks of health. In terms of congruence, Paul was able to look back on his life and affirm its value. This value came not only from his role as a physician, but also from his role as a father, a husband, a friend, and a community member. He was also able to look forward and find hope and meaning in his future, both in this life and beyond. He also then had coherence.

The community he served struggled with his illness more than he did. At one point, shortly after the initial diagnosis, friends decided that they needed to have a prayer vigil on his behalf. They made arrangements with the Presbyterian Church and held a 24-hour vigil, encouraging people to stop by the sanctuary and offer prayers for healing. Hundreds of people, out of a community of 2800 people, did. Amazingly, Paul's cancer went into remission. The tumor shrank, the pain subsided, and he was able to return to work for several years. Eventually the tumor did grow, and the pain and weakness returned, but this was not a big issue for Paul. He would laughingly call the remission his 'Lazarus experience,' referring to the man raised from death by Christ in the Gospels. 'Lazarus,' he noted, 'eventually died again. He just got some bonus time.' Paul considered this time of remission as bonus time, given to him by God so he could get closer to his family, take some special trips with his wife, and learn how much other people loved him.

When Paul died in 1985 an entire community joined together to celebrate a life well lived. Not only was the sanctuary full, but hundreds more watched the service via closed-circuit television. Was Paul cured? No. Did he find healing? Absolutely. Was he able to find joy, satisfaction, and purpose during his years of illness? 'In some ways,' he asserted before he died, 'these were some of the richest years of my life.'

Some people find cure. Some people find healing. Some find cure without healing. Some find healing without cure. The ultimate goal of healthcare should not be cure alone, but the healing of the whole person. The goal of the healer should be to work toward cure, within the context of healing. Cure of the body, and healing in every other facet of the self.

The goal of this book is to explore how that goal is reached.

Questions for reflection

- What is the difference between 'cure' and 'healing'?
- How would you define health?
- How does your definition of health change or reinforce your concept of healing and healthcare?
- What is the role of the healer?

Notes

1   Stewart M, Brown JB, Weston WW, McWhinney IR, McWilliam C and Freeman TR (1995) *Patient Centered Medicine*. Sage Publications, Thousand Oaks, CA, pp.4–5 (Quoting Faber K *Nosography in Modern Internal Medicine* (Jean Marting (trans.)). Paul B Hoeber, New York, NY, p.35.)

2   Miller WR (ed.) (1999) *Integrating Spirituality into Treatment*. American Psychological Association, Washington DC.

3   Stewart M, Brown JB, Weston WW, McWhinney IR, McWilliam C and Freeman TR (1995) *Patient Centered Medicine*. Sage, Thousand Oaks, CA, pp.31–3.

4   Stewart M, Brown JB, Weston WW, McWhinney IR, McWilliam C and Freeman TR (1995) *Patient Centered Medicine*. Sage, Thousand Oaks, CA, p.41.

5   Harris RL, Arche GL Jr and Waltke B (1980) *Theological Wordbook of the Old Testament, Vol. I*. Moody Press, Chicago, IL, p.136.

6   Kittel GF (trans. Bromiley GE) (1971) *Theological Dictionary of the New Testament, Vol VII*. Eerdmans, Grand Rapids, MI, p.1048.

7   Kittel GF (trans. Bromiley GE) (1971) *Theological Dictionary of the New Testament, Vol VII*. Eerdmans, Grand Rapids, MI, p.1060.

8   Gehman HS (ed.) (1970) *The New Westminster Dictionary of the Bible*. Westminster Press, Philadelphia, PA, p.901.

9   Gehman HS (ed.) (1970) *The New Westminster Dictionary of the Bible*. Westminster Press, Philadelphia, PA, p.901.

10   Khan HI (1997) *The Inner Life*. Shambhala Publications, Boston, MA, p.18.

11   Khan HI (1997) *The Inner Life*. Shambhala Publications, Boston, MA, p.18.

12   Khan HI (1997) *The Inner Life*. Shambhala Publications, Boston, MA, p.8.

13   Smith H (1965) *The Religions of Man*. Harper & Row, Perennial Library, NY, p.125.

14   Humphries C (1951) *Buddhism*. Pelican Books, Harmondsworth, England, p.91.

15   Quoted in Smith H (1965) *The Religions of Man*. Harper & Row, Perennial Library, NY, p.125.

16   Quoted in Smith H (1965) *The Religions of Man*. Harper & Row, Perennial Library, NY, p.129.

17   Quoted in Smith H (1965) *The Religions of Man*. Harper & Row, Perennial Library, NY, p.131.

18   Tournier P (1964) *The Whole Person in a Broken World*. Harper & Row, NY, p.36.

19   Tournier P (1964) *The Whole Person in a Broken World*. Harper & Row, NY, p.41.

20   Carrel A (1935) *Man, the Unknown.* Harper & Row, NY.
21   de Rougemont J (1945) *Vie du corps et vie des nerveux.* Editions du Rhone, Geneva, as quoted in Tournier P (1964) *The Whole Person in a Broken World.* Harper & Row, NY, pp.50–1.
22   Tournier P (1964) *The Whole Person in a Broken World.* Harper & Row, NY, p.52.
23   Satir V (1972) *Peoplemaking.* Science and Behavior Books, Inc., Palo Alto, CA, p.3.
24   Koenig HG (1994) *Aging and God.* The Haworth Press, Binghamton, NY; Roberts JA *et al.* (1997) *Journal of Obstetrics and Gynecology.* **176**(1): 166–72; McNeill JA *et al.* (1998) *Journal of Pain and Symptom Management.* **16**(1): 29–40.
25   Zinnbauer BJ *et al.* (1997) Religions and spirituality: unfuzzying the fuzzy. *Journal for the Scientific Study of Religion.* **36**(4): 549–64.
26   Developed by a group of medical students participating in an elective on Spirituality and Medicine at Oregon Health and Science University, 2000, Stephen Kliewer, D.Min Course Director.
27   Miller WR (ed.) (1999) *Integrating Spirituality into Treatment.* American Psychological Association, Washington DC.
28   *Webster's Dictionary* (1980).
29   Larson DB, Swyers JP and McCullough ME (eds) (1997) *Scientific Research on Spirituality and Health: a consensus report.* National Institute of Healthcare Research, Rockville, MD.
30   Zinnbauer BJ *et al.* (1997) Religions and spirituality: unfuzzying the fuzzy. *Journal for the Scientific Study of Religion.* **36**(4): 549–64.
31   Thoreson CE (1998) Spirituality, health and science: the coming revival? In: S Roth-Roemer, S Kurpius Robinson and C Carmin (eds) *The Emerging Role of Counseling Psychology in Health Care.* Norton, New York, pp.409–31, as referenced in Miller WR (ed.) (1999) *Integrating Spirituality into Treatment.* American Psychological Association, Washington DC.
32   Matthews DA with Clark C (1998) *The Faith Factor.* Viking, New York, NY, p.18.
33   Koenig HG, McCullough ME and Larson DB (2001) *Handbook of Religion and Health.* Oxford University Press, Oxford, p.19.
34   Hinterkopf E (1998) *Integrating Spirituality in Counseling.* American Counseling Association, Alexandria, VA, p.10.
35   Hinterkopf E (1998) *Integrating Spirituality in Counseling.* American Counseling Association, Alexandria, VA, p.11.
36   Nouwen H (1975) *Reaching Out.* Doubleday, New York, NY.
37   Rapgay L (1996) *The Tibetan Book of Healing.* Passage Press, Salt Lake City, UT, p.15.
38   Rapgay L (1996) *The Tibetan Book of Healing.* Passage Press, Salt Lake City, UT, p.15.
39   Miller WR (ed.) (1999) *Integrating Spirituality into Treatment.* American Psychological Association, Washington DC, p.4.
40   Miller WR (ed.) (1999) *Integrating Spirituality into Treatment.* American Psychological Association, Washington DC, p.5.
41   Walther DA (1987) *Frameworks: patterns for living and believing today.* Pilgrim, New York, NY, p.16–33.
42   Originally published in *Perspectives on Business Innovation.* Published on KurzweilAI. net, May 1, 2003. www.kurzweilai.net/articles/art0563.html.
43   Originally published in *Perspectives on Business Innovation.* Published on KurzweilAI. net, May 1, 2003. www.kurzweilai.net/articles/art0563.html.
44   Miller WR (ed.) (1999) *Integrating Spirituality into Treatment.* American Psychological Association, Washington DC, p.5.

CHAPTER 2

Toward a model of integration

Science without religion is lame,
religion without science is blind.
                    Albert Einstein, *Philosophy and Religion*, 1941

The relationship of healing to spirituality has been both long and varied. The roots of medicine are deeply imbedded in spirituality, with spiritual leaders being some of the earliest 'healers.' Indeed the relationship of medicine and spirituality was seen as not only positive and synergistic, but essential and inherent. But with the advent of the age of reason and the accompanying scientific revolution, the relationship between spirituality and medicine changed, from one of alliance to one of enmity.

A chasm is born

The radical shift in paradigms represented by this 'revolution' began in the late 1500s and was due to the influence of philosopher/scientists such as Bacon, Voltaire, and Descartes. René Descartes was born in 1596 in Touraine, France, where his father was a Councillor of the Brittany Parliament. Descartes was placed in Jesuit school and thus received his formal education from the Church. After a few years of legal studies, and one year of military service, Descartes turned his attention to the questions of philosophy. His efforts were heavily influenced by Isaac Beeckman, a student of sciences he met while serving in the army of Maurice of Nassau. In a letter written in March of 1619 he declared that his goal in life was 'to give the public ... an entirely new science ... so that almost nothing will remain to be discovered in geometry.'[1] He spent nine years developing and testing the principles of a new logic-based approach to human knowledge. In 1628 Descartes attended a conference held in Paris and listened to a discourse refuting the Aristotelian teaching then dominant in the schools. Descartes found himself in disagreement with the speaker Chandoux, who had argued that probability is the lone basis on which true knowledge can be based. Descartes rose and offered his own thesis, that certainty, not probability, is the only basis on which knowledge can be based.

His method, which drew heavily from the world of mathematics, had two simple requirements:

1 that we start from what is so simple and evident as to be unquestionable and
2 that we advance from the simple to the complex, taking no step which is not equally incontestable.

As he notes in his treatise, aptly titled 'The Discourse on Method,' 'I came to believe that the four following rules would be found sufficient, always provided I took the firm and unswerving resolve never in a single instance to fail in observing them.'[2]

His four rules, which clearly reflect the two principles he put forth in Paris, can be summarized as follows.

1   Accept nothing as true which one does not know, based on evidence, to be such.
2   Divide each of the difficulties or problems examined into as many parts as may be required for its adequate solution.
3   Arrange one's thoughts in order, beginning with the things simplest and easiest to know, so that one may move, step by step, to the more complex.
4   In all cases make enumerations so complete and reviews so general as to be assured of missing nothing.[3]

Descartes believed that his principles applied both to animate and inanimate nature and he clearly understood the impact these principles would have on medicine. Norman Kemp Smith notes that Descartes believed that 'it would be in medicine, even more than in mechanics, that his most important and beneficent discoveries would be made. For if all bodily processes are mechanistically caused, bodily diseases, once their causes have been determined, should be remediable with the same precision and certainty as the disorders of a clock.'[4]

Francis Bacon also contributed significantly to the transformation taking place in the world of science. Bacon was a man of great capacity, a true Renaissance man, who, although frail and often ill, successfully pursued an incredible range of interests and careers. He was a jurist, courtier, parliamentarian, writer, and philosopher. Although he is best known today for his philosophical writings, he was extremely active in the world of politics, having a long and honorable career in Parliament, and being a Counsel to the Court of England (Queen Elizabeth I and King James I). Bacon, like Descartes, believed that in order for people to gain new knowledge it would be necessary to totally reconstruct the sciences and build human knowledge on the proper foundation. Bacon conceived an approach for reconstruction and divided his effort into six parts. Of these only two, *The Divisions of the Sciences* and *The New Organon*, were developed fully. Bacon's main principles were similar to those of Descartes, and his methodology was intended to be empirical and inductive, as opposed to the prevailing scholastic method of his time, which was deductive and syllogistic.

Bacon's method involved three distinct steps. The first step is to become familiar with the facts surrounding the object of investigation. Second, one engages in a process of exclusion and rejection using reason to analyze the facts and eliminate unrelated elements. From the remaining facts one develops basic axioms. These axioms are repeatedly tested, and those that 'pass' the test become general principles or truths. Bacon and Descartes agreed that securing knowledge meant moving from the lesser to the greater, from the particular to the general. The key to the process is the mandate to check and recheck the facts.

Bacon had a unique style and enjoyed contracting his thoughts into short statements or aphorisms. His method is revealed in the aphorisms that make up much of the *New Organon*.

> Man, being the servant and interpreter of Nature, can do and understand so much only as he has observed in fact or through the course of nature; beyond this he neither knows anything nor can do anything.
>
> Human knowledge and human power meet in one, for where the cause is not known, the effect cannot be produced. Nature to be commanded must be obeyed...

The logic in use now serves rather to fix and give stability to the errors which have their foundation in commonly received motions than to help the search after truth.[5]

The work of people such as Descartes and Bacon became the foundation for what we now call the scientific method, the systematic examination of empirical data using a rational and scientific approach to knowledge. In medicine we see the methodologies propounded by these writers put into practice by people such as Laennec,[6] who said one must observe carefully for causation of disease, identify the physiological issue clearly, and then introduce an appropriate intervention. He insisted that in order to verify that the intervention is effective the impact of that intervention must be observed and documented. The intervention must be repeated and observed multiple times and in multiple circumstances with the goal of clearly establishing a pattern of effect. By the 1600s this new scientific method was well established and it was being used to develop new medical theories.

However, since this new experimental method could not readily or confidently be applied to God or to one's experiences with God, religion/spirituality began to be separated from science, and a chasm developed between spirituality/religion and science/medicine. This chasm was widened by the tendency of the religious community to be a defender of the status quo and to reject many of the new discoveries that emerged as a result of the application of this scientific method. In 1633, for example, learning of the Inquisition's condemnation of Galileo's astronomy, Descartes suppressed his almost completed treatise *Le Monde*, the result of five years of study, and began to share his concepts in ways he felt were more acceptable to the Church. However, his books *Meditations*, which he wrote as an attempt to enlist the support of religious leaders, and *Principles* were both criticized severely by church scholars. Eventually Descartes gave up hope of finding general acceptance from the church and began to write with more openness. Many see the inflexibility of religious dogma in Descartes' time as continuing today, and as a factor hindering the integration of medicine and spirituality.

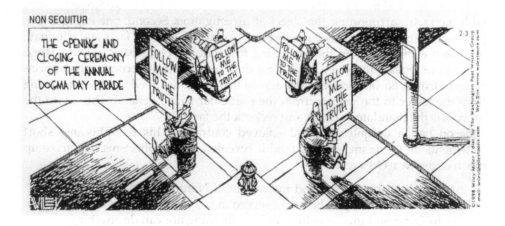

Figure 2.1

Non Sequitur © 1998 Wiley Miller. Distributed by Universal Press Syndicate, Inc. Reprinted with permission. All rights reserved.

The gap between spirituality and science, religion, and medicine continued to widen as, over the years, there has been an ever-increasing emphasis on the science of medicine, created by an exponential growth of scientific knowledge relevant to medical practice. The public's increased demand for technologically sophisticated medical care has intensified as scientific advances have been broadcast through television, newspapers, magazines, and more recently the internet. Within the medical community itself there has been an increased emphasis on tools such as evidence-based medicine, and medical practice has become centered on the task of choosing treatments proved effective through rigorous study.[7] The unfortunate result has been the neglect of those aspects of the 'art of medicine' that do not fall naturally into the realm of the scientific.

There have always been voices that have argued against this neglect. Early on many deeply spiritual scientists such as Pascal[8] struggled to keep the world of science and the world of faith connected, and more recently people such as Herbert Benson MD of Harvard[9] and Jim Gordon MD of the Center for Mind Body Medicine[10] have spoken about an important and positive connection between spirituality and medicine.

In spite of these efforts, however, spirituality has traditionally been shunned by the medical community. One problem is that it is inherently difficult to define spirituality, which cannot be easily quantified.[11] Attempts at definition are varied and distressingly vague for the scientific mind. This vagueness makes it extremely difficult to design credible studies that accurately assess the role of spirituality in health and healing. Yet without such studies physicians, rooted in the scientific method, are hesitant to integrate this component into clinical practice. Generally speaking, those studies attempting to assess the impact of spirituality on health have focused on religious practices such as worship or prayer, since these activities can be easily observed and quantified. Intensifying the distrust generated by the diaphanous nature of spirituality are such factors as dogmatic hostility and the misuse and abuse of religion. When these factors are added to the inability to quantify spirituality, distrust evolves into dislike.

As a result, many reputable health professionals have seen religious practice as something negative that adversely affects patients. Mandel, in *The Psychobiology of Consciousness*, calls spirituality a 'temporal lobe dysfunction.'[12] Perhaps a more egregious example was the use of spirituality in the DMS III R Glossary of Technical Terms. In that document all allusions to spirituality were illustrations of psychopathology. It is interesting to note that 22.2% of the negative illustrations in that version of the glossary had religious content, while none had sexual, ethnic, racial, or cultural content. In one of the more famous condemnations of religion, Freud, in his book *Future of an Illusion*, noted that 'Religion would thus be the universal obsessional neurosis of humanity.'[13] Wendell Watters, a physician and Professor of Psychiatry at McMaster University in Ontario, Canada, insisted, 'religion is not only irrelevant but actually harmful to human beings ...'[14] Albert Ellis, founder of the Rational Emotive Therapy Institute in New York, wrote in 1980 that, 'Devout orthodox or dogmatic religion is significantly correlated with emotional disturbance.'[15] In the *Handbook of Religion and Health* the authors list a number of behaviors resulting from religious involvement that have a potential negative impact on health.[16] In most cases these behaviors involve a failure to use or comply with traditional medical care. In some cases, however, the list shifts from 'sins of omission' to 'sins of commission' and involve destructive behaviors that injure the self or others. The list includes the following activities:

- stopping life-saving medication
- failing to seek timely medical care
- refusing blood transfusions
- refusing childhood immunizations
- refusing prenatal care and physician-assisted delivery
- fostering child abuse
- withholding medical care for children
- religious abuse
- replacing mental healthcare with religion.

Some research supports the medical community's apprehension concerning the impact of religious beliefs. For example, some studies show a positive correlation between religiousness and such factors as prejudice, anxiety, depression, dependency, and social and community isolation.[17]

Thus, over the past several hundred years the relationship between medicine and religion became marginalized, and at times even toxic. The functional result of the chasm between the two was not so much overt antagonism, as an almost unconscious segmentation. The average physician simply did not consider religion as something to be considered within the context of healthcare. Eventually the world of spirituality and the world of medicine simply did not touch, except perhaps in the hearts and minds of patients and their families.

The relationship revisited

Recently there has been a shift of both public and professional sentiment toward the inclusion of spirituality in the practice of medicine. This shift has been fueled by a discussion of this topic in both popular and professional journals. In 1999, faculty at Oregon Health and Science University conducted a literature search of a large public library database of popular magazines. Using the key words 'spirituality' and 'health' they were able to find only 25 articles from 1990–1994 that addressed spirituality in the context of healthcare. However, a search of publications from 1995–1999 revealed 100 articles, an impressive increase. A parallel study of the medical literature showed a similar change. Searching MedLine using the keyword 'spirituality' produced 52 articles from 1960–1990, 90 from 1991–1995, and almost 200 from 1996–1999.[18] A more recent search produced 554 citations from January 2000 to April 2003.

Impetus from research

Much of the new interest in the relationship of spirituality and medicine has been the result of a group of physicians who have insisted that medical research shows religion to be a benefit not a hindrance to health. The late David Larson MD, MSPH of the International Center for the Integration of Health and Spirituality (ICIHS) and his collaborators performed an extensive review of journals identifying a large number of studies including spiritual indicators. This review showed a strong trend toward identifying spirituality as a positive factor in coping with illness, prevention of illness, and aiding in treatment.[19] Harold G Koenig of Duke University also explored the relationship between religion and health, concluding that the evidence from research, if looked at objectively, demonstrates a positive correlation between religion and health. His book asks the critical question, 'Is Religion Good for Your Health?',[20] and posits a positive answer. Recently Koenig helped develop the *Handbook of Religion and Health*,[21] which systematically reviews and rates research conducted on the relationship between religion and a variety of mental and physical health conditions up to the year 2000. In a majority of cases the impact of religion was found to be positive.

There are some very significant limitations, however, to the research that has been done. The very title of the *Handbook of Religion and Health* is informative. It uses the term 'religion,' rather than the term 'spirituality.' As we have discussed earlier, spirituality, which is defined many ways, is often seen as a search for what is sacred or holy in life, coupled with some kind of transcendent (beyond self) relationship with God or a higher power or universal energy.[22] Religion is more on prescribed beliefs, rituals, and practices as well as social institutional features.[23] This means that religion is more concrete than spirituality, and thus more quantifiable. The result is that most of the research done examines specific religious practices such as prayer and worship and how they impact health rather than at a person's spirituality. Only a relatively small percentage of studies involve an attempt to measure the spiritual wellness of the patient or ask people to self-rate the importance of faith in their lives. Another general characteristic of this body of research is that the focus is on the pre-existing religiosity or spirituality of the patients. Few studies have been done where a 'spiritual intervention' such as prayer has been introduced. For example, in the research inventory of 1600 studies at the end of the *Handbook* only 37 were Spiritual/Faith Healing or Prayer studies.

That being said, through the year 2000 over 1600 studies have been conducted that include a religious or spiritual component. This research can be broken down into three major categories: religion and mental health, religion and physical disorders, and religion and the use of health services. A smaller number of studies focus on research issues, spiritual development, and implications for health and religious professionals.

These studies are marked by a great deal of diversity. Although most studies in English have focused on 'Western faiths' such as Roman Catholicism, Orthodoxy, mainline and fundamentalist Protestantism, Pentecostalism, Jehovah's Witnesses, Judaism, and Mormonism, studies have also looked at such faiths as Baha'i, Hare Krishna, Islam, Sikhism, and Hinduism.[13,14] Geographic or national diversity is also present, with 39 different countries specifically listed as study locales and with many other studies listing 'world' as the locale. In some cases, especially in the area of mental health (depression and psychoses), type of religious affiliation did seem to be a factor in outcomes, both positive and negative.[24] Some studies actually compare a variety of nations, cultures, or faith systems, and in one study focusing on suicide, a difference in nationality and culture created totally opposite results.[25]

- **Religion and mental health:** Studies have examined the impact of religion or spirituality on well-being, self-esteem, depression, and suicide, as well as alcohol and drug use and abuse. Religious or spiritual people, especially those who are regularly involved with a community of faith, experience depression less often

Table 2.1 Areas of spirituality research to date

Major focus	Subtopics	Earliest publication	Number of publications
Mental health	Religious coping, hope and optimism, purpose/meaning in life, self-esteem, bereavement, social support, depression, suicide, assisted suicide/euthanasia, anxiety, schizophrenia/psychosis, alcohol use/abuse, drug use/abuse, delinquency/crime, marital instability, personality, general mental health	1932	1075
Physical health	Heart disease, hypertension, cerebrovascular disease, immune system, cancer risk, mortality, functional disability, pain and somatic symptoms, health behaviors, miscellaneous	1902	455
Use of health services	General medical services, mental health services, disease prevention, health responsibility, compliance	1960	53
Clinical implications and applications	Health professionals, religious professionals	1973	131
Research	Measurement	1967	40
Miscellaneous	Religious beliefs/behaviors, religious/faith development, religious conversion, spiritual/faith healing, prayer, death and dying, religious harm	1902	171

than others, are less likely to abuse drugs or alcohol, cope with life issues and illness more effectively, and are less likely to commit suicide.[12]

- **Religion and physical disorders:** Studies have focused specifically on the effect of faith on heart disease, hypertension, cerebrovascular disease, immune system dysfunctions, and cancer. Other studies have looked at broader issues such as pain and mortality.[12] Demonstrable results have included reduced hypertension,[16,17] better lipid profiles,[18,19] improved immune function,[20,21] and lower cholesterol levels[22] in persons who participate in religious activities and/or take spirituality seriously.

- **Religion and use of health services:** Research on the use of health services focuses on such matters as screening[23] and compliance.[24] One of the interesting factors here is the role of religion in non-compliance. The refusal of Jehovah's Witnesses to receive blood products has been a highly visible example, but other issues – more subtle, but nevertheless critical – emerge when one examines the literature. These include non-compliance due to a belief that a higher power 'caused' the illness, or that illness is the result of 'sinful' behavior.[25]

In general, research shows the impact of religion and spirituality on health outcomes, the ability of patients to cope, and the prevention of morbidity and

Table 2.2 Propositions regarding the effect of spirituality on physical outcomes

Proposition/Studies	Rating* (#/letter)
Religious coping aids stress management	
Ellison CG and Taylor RJ (1996) Turning to prayer: social and situational antecedents of religious coping among African Americans. *Rev Religious Research*. **38**: 111–31.	8/NA
Pargament KI, Smith BW, Koenig HG *et al*. (1998) Patterns of positive and negative religious coping with major life stressors. *J Scientific Study Religion*. **37**(4): 710–24.	8/NA
Spirituality/religious affiliation prevents substance abuse	
Bell R, Wechsler H and Johnston LD (1997) Correlates of college student marijuana use: results of a US national survey. *Addiction*. **92**: 571–81.	9/NA
Religious practices/spirituality decreases the incidence of depression	
Idler EL and Kasl S (1992) Religion, disability, depression, and the timing of death. *Am J Sociology*. **97**: 1052–79.	10/NA
Kennedy GJ, Kelman HR, Thomas C *et al*. (1996) The relation of religious preference and practice to depressive symptoms among 1855 older adults. *J Gerontol*. **51B**: 301–8.	10/NA
Religious practice/spirituality lowers suicide rates	
Neeleman J, Halpern D and Leon D (1997) Tolerance of suicide, religion, and suicide rates: an ecological and individual study in 19 Western countries. *Psychol Med*. **27**(5): 1165–71.	10/NA
Religious practice/spirituality prevents hypertension/lowers blood pressure	
Steffen PR, Hinderliter AL, Blumenthal JA *et al*. (2001) Religious coping, ethnicity, and ambulatory blood pressure. *Psychosomatic Med*. **63**: 523–30.	7/A–B
Koenig HG, George LK, Hays JC *et al*. (1998) The relationships between religious activities and blood pressure in older adults. *International J Psych Med*. **28**: 189–213.	9/A–B
Religious practice/spirituality is related to better lipid profiles	
Friedlander Y, Kark JD and Stein Y (1987) Religious observance and plasma lipids and lipoproteins among 17 year old Jewish residents of Jerusalem. *Prevent Med*. **16**: 70–9.	8/B
Religious practice/spirituality is associated with better immune function	
Woods TE, Antoni MH, Ironson GH *et al*. (1999) Religiosity is associated with affective and immune status in symptomatic HIV-infected gay men. *J Psychosomatic Research*. **46**: 165–76.	7/B
Koenig HG, Cohen JH, George LK *et al*. (1997) Attendance at religious services, interleukin-6, and other biological parameters of immune function in older adults. *International J Psych Med*. **27**: 233–50.	8/A–B
Religious practice/spirituality is related to lower cholesterol	
Patel C, Marmot MG, Terry DJ *et al*. (1985) Trial of relaxation in reducing coronary risk: Four year follow up. *BMJ*. **290**: 1103–6.	NA/A
Attendance at church services leads to longer life	
Koenig JG, Hays JC, Larson DB *et al*. Does religious attendance prolong survival? A six-year follow-up study of 3,968 older adults. *J Gerontology Series A: Biologic Sci Med Sci*. **54A**: M370–6.	9/A

= Rating system from Koenig *et al*., *Handbook of Religion and Health*. Scale of 1–10 (1=poor, 10=excellent). Based on overall study design, sampling method, quality of religious measure, quality of statistical analysis, interpretation of results, and discussion in the context of existing literature. Methodology validated by outside reviewers.

Letter = Rating system from Miller WR and Thoresen CE, *Spirituality, Religion and Health: an emerging research field*. A = Methodologically Sound, B = Methodologically Sound with at least one methodological limitation, NA = not rated by this system.

mortality is positive. Of those studies reviewed in the *Handbook*, where the impact of spirituality could be classified as positive, negative, no association, complex, or mixed, 70% showed a positive impact (68% a strong positive with p<0.05) while only 5% showed a negative impact. The studies show that spirituality and religion benefit patients by helping prevent illness, increasing[26] the ability to cope, and improving outcomes.

It is important to note that in spite of this positive trend there are times when the research indicates a negative impact. A recent article in *American Psychologist* notes there is more evidence that religion or spirituality impedes recovery than that it improves recovery.[22] It is important to note that the outcome cited by the article was connected to religious struggle or to negative coping (e.g., 'I feel God has abandoned me'). With this focus the result is not surprising and it underscores the need to support positive religious coping and to help patients move beyond negative religious coping. This evidence is also a reminder that spirituality can be either healthy or pathological. Indeed it is probably better, when thinking about spirituality in the healthcare context, to think about whether the spirituality is healthy or unhealthy, rather than whether spirituality is present or absent. Everyone has a spirituality of some sort. How that spirituality impacts the other aspects of the self, and whether that impact is positive or negative are the real issues.

Impetus from patient need

Another factor driving the interest in the integration of spirituality and medicine is patient interest and need. According to myriad surveys, most Americans consider spirituality and religion a significant part of who they are.[27] Research in the field indicates that spirituality and religion are seen as a core aspect of life, and patients want physicians to address them as whole human beings rather than as purely physical machines.[28] A public survey done in 1996 by *USA Weekend* showed that 63% of patients believe doctors should ask about spirituality issues, but only 10% of the respondents have actually been asked.[29] In another study, 77% of patients surveyed said physicians should consider patients' spiritual needs, and 37% wanted physicians to discuss religious beliefs with them more frequently.[30]

Questions for reflection

- How do you feel about the integration of medicine and spirituality?
- What are, for you, the most compelling reasons for the integration of spirituality into treatment?
- Have you ever (as a physician or a patient) participated in a therapeutic encounter where spirituality was addressed?
- What was the impact of that experience?

Point, counter-point

In spite of the movement toward integration, the emergence of certain major issues has caused people to rethink the connection between medicine and spirituality. Studies show a gap between patient expectation and physician practice in this area. Patients seem to desire integration, but, in spite of the fact that physicians as a group 'reported strong religious or spiritual orientation,' such integration hasn't occurred.[31] In short, physician interest in spirituality on the personal level has not been translated into practice behaviors. The reluctance of physicians to integrate spirituality into practice corresponds with a wide range of concerns expressed by physicians in a number of recent surveys.[32] The list of concerns elicited by Mark Ellis, Daniel C Vinson, and Bernard Ewigman, clearly highlights the kinds of barriers facing those physicians who wish to address spirituality in the clinical relationship.[33] According to the physicians surveyed, integration was hindered by those factors listed in Box 2.1.

Box 2.1 Barriers to integration

- Lack of time – 71%
- Lack of experience/training – 59%
- Uncertainty about how to identify patients who desire a discussion of spiritual issues – 56%
- Concern that the physician will project his or her own beliefs – 52%
- Uncertainty about how to manage spiritual issues raised by patients – 48.8%
- Belief that spiritual issues must take a lower priority than more acute medical issues – 45.3%
- Belief that expressing spiritual concerns is not appropriate to the physician's role – 31%
- Belief that patients do not want to share spiritual concerns with the physician – 29.5%
- Lack of continuity in relationship with patients – 27.2%
- Difficulty of using appropriately understood language in discussion of spiritual issues – 23.8%
- Negative attitudes of peers toward spiritual assessment of patients – 22.9%

It is interesting that the top three concerns seem to be practical rather than philosophical or ethical. The most critical barrier is time, followed by training and competence. The first 'ethical' issue to be listed is that of imposing one's own belief inappropriately, or the issue of proper relationship boundaries. For the most part the physicians involved in this study (69%) did not see the validity of integration as the issue but instead had concerns related to the practical issue of how such integration might occur in a practical and appropriate manner.

Recently, however, a group of articles have been published which strongly challenge the entire premise of integration. Richard P Sloan and his associates, in the 'Sounding Board' section of the *New England Journal of Medicine*, state that they are 'troubled by the uncritical embrace of this trend...'[34] They cite a number of reasons to be wary of this integration.

1 Studies suggesting a relationship between spirituality and health are flawed.
2 The unique nature of the patient/physician relationship causes physician assumptions and beliefs to have undue influence.
3 Physicians have no expertise in spiritual matters.
4 Most patients do not truly want to discuss spiritual issues, and interest does not necessarily justify the incorporation of religious matters.
5 The integration of spirituality into practice is an attempt to use religion that trivializes a deep and complex reality.

A similar article in *The Lancet* echoed these same concerns.[29] Again the empirical evidence is challenged, and a variety of ethical concerns are added.

The first ethical issue relates to relationship boundaries. The authors insist that 'when doctors depart from areas of established expertise to promote a non-medical agenda, they abuse their status as professionals.' At the root of this concern is the presence of a 'power differential' between physicians and a majority of their patients. Physicians have a unique body of knowledge inaccessible to most people. They function in a unique, mysterious, and often frightening (to the patient) environment. They are given an incredible amount of power by patients. Add to these factors the essential vulnerability of a person who is ill and the fact that many people are very suggestible when they are ill. All of this creates a tremendous potential for abuse. Critics of the integration of spirituality and medicine believe that when physicians address spiritual issues with patients they may be 'taking advantage' of them to further their own agendas. The second issue involves the ethics of 'taking into account' spiritual issues versus 'taking them on' as the objects of interventions. A third ethical problem focuses on the possibility that physicians might actually do harm to patients by linking health status and spirituality.[35]

Key issues for integration

The cautions put forth by these writers are worthy of serious consideration. They highlight a number of issues that must be addressed if we are to develop a responsible model of integration.

Quality of the research

The first issue centers on the research that has been used to justify integration. Certainly there is a need for added and improved research on the impact of religion and spirituality on health. Koenig and his collaborators rate only 18.5% of the studies an 8, 9, or 10, on a quality scale of 1 to 10 (with 10 being excellent) and assert that 'we have only scratched the surface in acquiring knowledge about the influences of religion on health, the influences of health on religion, and the mechanisms by which these effects occur.'[36] A more recent review of studies attempting to link religiosity to physiological processes notes that the results are 'suggestive,' but cites the need for additional research that combines stronger research methodology with more representative populations.[37] In sum, evidence from the research is neither strong enough to validate the move toward integration, nor weak enough to invalidate it. An effective model of integration can be justified by the research, but this must be done cautiously.

Use or misuse of spirituality

This leads to the second major issue, the way spirituality is applied or used in the therapeutic process. Those who focus on the research point out that many studies suggest that spirituality/religion is helpful in terms of prevention, outcome, and coping. Religion, as Koenig suggests in his title, might well be 'good for your health.' If one has an active spiritual life, prays, or worships, the research does suggest that illness is less frequent, recovery is faster, coping is more effective during periods of illness. During a talk on medicine and spirituality at Oregon Health and Science University some facts were presented on the impact of faith on health.[38] A series of research projects were highlighted, including the 1988 study by RC Byrd on the positive therapeutic effects of intercessory prayer in a coronary care unit population. In this study it was shown that intercessory prayer, offered by a third party, improved the outcomes for patients admitted to a coronary care unit in San Francisco.[39] The study was well designed.

- The study took 393 patients hospitalized in the coronary care unit of San Francisco General Hospital.
- Byrd, a cardiologist, randomly split the patients into two groups.
- 192 patients received intercessory prayer by Christian prayer groups located outside the hospital.
- 201 patients (the control group) received no prayer by the groups.
- This was a double blind study. Neither the patients nor their physicians knew which patients had prayers offered on their behalf.

The results, ascertained through a retroactive chart review were statistically significant.

Table 2.3   Outcome of Byrd study

New problems or events	Prayer	Control
Congestive heart failure	4	10
Cardiopulmonary arrest	3	8
Pneumonia	2	7
Antibiotics needed	2	7
Diuretics needed	2	9
Good track (no new diagnosis/therapy)	85%	73%
Bad track (high morbidity risk/died)	14%	22%

Fewer complications and less need for secondary interventions occurred with the prayer group than with the control group. From the perspective of whether they followed a 'good track' or a 'bad track,' there was a 12% improvement among those who had been the subject of intercessory prayer. Once this information was provided to the medical students the suggestion was made that, based on such an improvement, spirituality ought to be taken seriously in treatment. During a question and answer period following the lecture one of the medical students expressed reservations. His comment to the speaker made everyone think. 'I do not think,' he asserted, 'that it is helpful to show that God is 12% more effective than a placebo.' He was not questioning the validity of the study and he was not really questioning whether integrating spirituality and medicine was appropriate. Rather he was challenging the use of spirituality in this manner.

What is the appropriate role of spirituality or religion in healing? Is it proper to approach spirituality the same way one approaches a new medical/scientific intervention? Can faith be used the same way a drug is used? Can we say, 'Take two prayers and see me in the morning?' It is an important theological question. Koenig titles one of his books *The Healing Power of Faith: how belief and prayer can help you triumph over disease.*[40] The implications of the title are clear. Dale Matthews in his book *The Faith Factor* overtly presents religious involvement as an intervention that can be used for the benefit of health. He presents a scenario in which a patient has a severe medical problem, chest pains. The doctor, after reviewing the results of an angiogram, recommends bypass surgery. In response to the patient's inquiry about how best to prepare for the surgery, the physician says, 'I just finished reading an article in a medical journal that described one factor that will lead to a better recovery. Would you like to know what it is?' Matthews concludes, 'It's hard to imagine [the patient] saying "no," isn't it?'[41]

From a theological perspective such an approach is disturbing because it suggests a direct cause and effect relationship between religious practice and health. This is much the same as suggesting there is a direct cause and effect relationship between sin and illness. While it is clear that faith may have an impact on health, to imply this kind of causality is theologically marginal. Faith is no guarantee of health. Faithfulness does not necessarily lead to what is generally perceived as success. From the Christian tradition, examples of Paul and Job abound. The entire book of Job deals with the case of a man who, although faithful, is repeatedly afflicted with tragedy. Paul, the most powerful leader in the early Christian church, was afflicted with a 'thorn', a physical ailment, which in spite of his faith, was not healed (II Corinthians 12:7–10). As Jean-Claude Larchet notes in his book *The Theology of Illness*, 'there is no necessary relationship between the health of the body and the health of the soul.'[42] This statement is even more powerful since it comes from a theological perspective (Orthodox) that takes the impact of sin on human life very seriously. Yet even Larchet understands that it is theologically unsound to create a necessary relationship between health (or illness) and a lack or presence of faith.

One of the major problems is that such an approach may create a scenario where the sacred or divine is 'obligated' to prevent illness, or facilitate healing. Normally this concept is linked with a prerequisite faith or faithfulness. If a person has enough faith or has been obedient (behaviorally) enough to the divine, then they can ask God to bring cure into their lives, and God will do it. In some cases, people feel God will be 'inclined' to generate healing, but in other cases people feel God 'must' offering healing. If one carries this concept to its logical conclusion then one must believe that a failure to receive healing or blessing must indicate either a lack of faith or the presence of sin. Either way a failure to receive the benefit of healing by necessity indicates failure on the part of the believer. Such a belief badly misconstrues the relationship between faith and illness.

In one small rural hospital a young pregnant woman arrived in great distress. Within a short period of time she experienced a spontaneous abortion. After two days she still remained in the hospital. Her overall physical condition was not good and she continued to experience a significant degree of hemorrhaging. Her physicians could not discern a biological reason why she should be having so much difficulty. Finally a local pastor was able to get her to share her story. The member of a small independent church, she had been visited by the 'elders' of her faith community. They, in talking to her about her miscarriage, had insisted that, since God would have healed her if she had been in a 'right relationship,' she must have been sinful and deserved the tragedy that had befallen her.

This story does not illustrate the views of people such as Koenig and Matthews, but it does illustrate the danger of suggesting a cause and effect relationship between faith and health. While we can suggest that faith is beneficial, we must be very careful not to create a simplistic formula that does more harm than good. Any model for integration must avoid strategies that 'use' faith and violates the nature, the complexity, and the depth of faith.

Perhaps the fundamental problem with focusing on spirituality as a therapeutic tool is that it may well ignore the essential nature of spirituality. Why do we pursue spirituality? This question is very difficult to answer, and there are probably as many answers as there are people, for spirituality is a very personal thing. For some the motivation for embracing spirituality may be escapist. People joke about people who see faith as 'fire insurance,' a way of avoiding punishment, including incarceration in hell after death, but there is no question that this is a motivation for many. Others use faith not to avoid 'unfortunate events' but to obtain personal benefit or gain. The perceived benefit can take many forms, including financial success, success in business or other endeavors, and an ability to find meaning and purpose in life. Neither the desire to escape the negative nor the hope to embrace benefit is inherently invalid, for spirituality clearly addresses both our fears and our hopes, but both desires can become unhealthy (spiritually speaking) if they become the single point of focus.

For others, spirituality is a way of chastening the soul or spirit, the way of discipline. It is a medium for shaping the self, for ordering life in a manner that meets the demands of the divine. Zossima, in Dostoevsky's book *The Brothers Karamazov*, gives eloquent voice to this perspective when he says, 'each of us is responsible before all, for everyone and for everything.'[43] This spirituality of responsibility is very pervasive and has a great impact both on lifestyle and attitude.

If spirituality is primarily a way to avoid the negative or gain benefit, then 'spirituality as a drug' might seem acceptable. However, many people have a concept of spirituality that does not allow for its simplistic 'use' in the healing process. A good example is Caroline Myss, a popular author who speaks of seven stages through which people must pass in order to obtain spiritual maturity. From these stages, which she draws from three spiritual traditions – the Hindus chakras, the Christian sacraments, and the Jewish Kabbalah's Tree of Life – Myss develops the seven sacred truths of the body and spirit. These truths provide insight into the goals of spirituality and reshape our thinking about the integration of spirituality and health. The seven truths, found in her book *Anatomy of the Spirit*, are as follows:[44]

1 All is One
2 Honor One Another

3 Honor Oneself
4 Love is Divine Power
5 Surrender Personal Will to Divine Will
6 Seek Only the Truth
7 Live in the Present Moment.

The first three truths relate primarily to relationships. Through spirituality one seeks to develop 'right' relationships, to the community (All is One), to significant others (Honor One Another), and with one's self (Honor Oneself). A right relationship is not only one in which one finds pleasure, satisfaction, or benefit, but one in which one gives these same gifts. It is being, relationally, a person who is capable of both receiving and giving. It is being both dependent and dependable, strong and weak, respected and respectful. These three truths point toward the goal of being a people who are at peace with themselves, and who bring benefit to those who come into their sphere.

Myss sees the fourth stage as the place where the mind and the spirit interface and the focus is heavily emotional. This truth, that love is divine power, has to do with motivation. Why do we seek right relationships? Because of love! We need, she asserts, 'to act out of love and compassion and recognize that the most powerful energy we have is love.'[45] Obviously the issue of motivation is significant. A motivation of love creates a far different dynamic than the motivation of power, or benefit.

According to the fifth truth, a person who seeks to be spiritual desires beyond all else 'the full release of [our] personal will into the "hands of the Divine".'[46] This is the same truth reflected in the Christian scriptures by such phrases as 'Thy will be done' (Matthew 6:10).

The sixth truth (Seek Only the Truth) relates to that facet of the person called the 'mind' or 'psyche.' A person pursues spirituality because he/she wants to know the truth, to connect with what is real. Often, in spiritual literature this desire for truth is connected with the concept of wisdom. A spiritual person seeks not only to know the truth, but to change, to shape his/her life according to that truth. This means that wisdom, or truth, is not always comfortable or easy, for at times the truth sears and chastens. It asks people to make changes that are painful, frightening, difficult, while leading those who seek it to new growth.

The final truth is 'Live in the Present Moment.' This truth relates to what is usually called the spirit and is relational in the sense that it refers to our relationship with the sacred, the divine. To live in the moment is to live connected, in an intimate and transcendent way, to that which is greater than one's self. This connection is the ultimate goal of spirituality – and it endows our lives with power and meaning. It is through this connection that energy and wisdom flow. A life in which this connection exists is, as noted above, not always comfortable or peaceful, often quite the opposite. The answers that are received may not always be the ones desired and the insights may be an imperative for change.

If we have a spirituality where the ultimate goal is a connection to the sacred or divine, that is truth revealing, transforming, a force for personal change, and an impetus for good, then can we approach spirituality and health in a manner that 'uses' spirituality as a medication? From this perspective such a use of spirituality seems inappropriate. This is not to say that the idea of healing is precluded. Instead it should be seen as a potential, though not inevitable, and natural consequence of an authentic spirituality.

Boundaries

A third issue that must be addressed is that of boundaries. Even the most enthusiastic proponents of integration are aware of the difficulties which arise in this arena.[47] One of the reasons this is so critical is because of the potential power differential between the physician and the patient. The issue of power, which we discussed briefly earlier, is a critical factor in any human relationship. Tony Campolo, a professor of sociology-anthropology, asserts that 'human beings hunger for power.' Friederich Nietzche argued that this hunger is the essence of our humanity, that 'the will to power' is the basic human drive.[48] Campolo defines power as 'the prerogative to determine what happens and the coercive force to make others yield to your wishes – even against their own will.'[49] Power can come from many sources. Money, knowledge, position, physical strength, situational dynamics, even love can give one person power over another. In Western culture there is a large 'power gap' between patients and physicians. This gap is economic and educational. It is also situational, with the patient, who has a great deal at stake, health and perhaps even life itself, being placed in an alien environment full of frightening technology, mysterious terminology, and dehumanizing starkness. It is cultural, with physicians being endowed by society in general with a significant amount of authority. Although an article a number of years ago declared that 'Dr God is dead,' there is still a tendency on the part of many patients to give physicians incredible power. It is this tendency that leads advertising agencies to continue to insist that products are 'doctor recommended.'

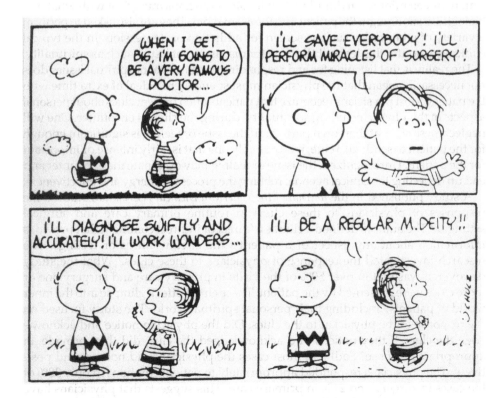

Figure 2.2

Peanuts © United Feature Syndicate, Inc.

Because the physician's words are given so much credence, physicians must use great caution when they move into the realm of opinion, value, or belief. As Post, Pulchaski, and Larson note, 'Adding a sacred or religious mystique to the power of the physician is suspect... Clearly it is important to delineate professional boundaries.'[50] The conclusion of these authors, who are strong proponents of the integration of medicine and spirituality, is that this integration of medicine and spirituality must always be focused on the patient's spirituality. It is appropriate for physicians to screen for spirituality and respect it. It is not appropriate for physicians to use their own spirituality as the basis for addressing spirituality in treatment. The authors note that: 'Patients should be permitted to express their spirituality, should they wish to, in a respectful and supportive clinical environment. It would, however, be disrespectful and not beneficial or supportive of autonomy to encourage patients to 'get religious or spiritual beliefs if they do not have them.'[51] In summation, any model of integration must take into account the differential of power, and build in safeguards to ensure that the patient is protected from the inappropriate use of power.

Time

A fourth issue that must be addressed, and the most common barrier cited by physicians for not integrating medicine and spirituality, is a lack of time. In today's practices physicians are increasingly pressured to be more time efficient and see more patients each day. It is not uncommon for the standard appointment time to be a mere fifteen minutes in duration. Obviously physicians must deal with whatever biological issue brought the patient into the exam room. They are also asked to perform a variety of other tasks, such as screen for addiction or depression. In the typical clinical encounter this leaves little time for discussion of issues such as spirituality.

The reality is that listening for and responding to emotional or spiritual issues does not necessarily mean that the physician must spend a great deal of extra time with the patient. Most physicians recognize that patients often present clues about personal aspects of their lives, including spirituality, during the clinical encounter. One will neglect these clues at their own peril, for if the issue or feeling is significant enough for the patient to send out a clue, it is probably one that is fairly intense or important for the patient. Unrecognized, the issue or feeling may dominate the encounter and end up deflecting the clinical agenda, robbing the process of energy and effectiveness.

A study published in the *Journal of the American Medical Association* studied the responses of physicians to these clues in routine primary care and surgical settings.[52] The authors defined a clue as a 'direct or indirect comment that provides information about any aspect of a patient's life circumstances or feelings. The research investigated the response of physicians to these clues.' What the study discovered was that in over 50% of the visits in primary care and surgery one or more clues were presented by the patient. These clues 'offer a glimpse into the inner world of patients,' including their personal spiritual world. The study focused on the response of the physician to the clues. Did the physician notice and acknowledge the clue? If they noticed and acknowledged the clue, did they provide an appropriate response? Sadly, in most cases the physicians did not respond positively. The physicians responded appropriately to patient emotions in only 38% of the cases in surgery and 21% in primary care. This suggests that physicians have room to improve in their ability to respond to patient clues.

One important component of this study was the exploration of the length of visit. As noted earlier, many physicians cite a lack of time as a major barrier to the integration of spirituality and medicine. They insist that if they acknowledge and respond to clues about emotional, spiritual, or social issues, they will not be able to complete the visit in a timely manner. This study found that 'the visit length both in primary care and in surgery was shortest when physicians made at least one positive response compared with when they missed the opportunity or when the patient repeatedly brought up the clue.' It appears that when physicians hear and respond to patients' expressed feelings and concerns, they can provide a benefit to the patient, create a stronger patient–physician relationship, and facilitate a more effective clinical encounter.

There are multiple benefits to the patient when the physician is willing to listen for and respond to the clues. First, the person feels heard, which is therapeutic in itself. Second, by using good communication skills the physician can help the patient become aware of, or even understand, feelings and issues that previously were unidentified or misunderstood. Thus by listening, physicians help move the patient to self-revelation and understanding. Third, the conversation provides the opportunity for the physicians to act as a catalyst for healing around whatever issue is discussed. This interchange conducted properly 'will help deepen the therapeutic alliance that is at the heart of clinical care.' Finally, listening and responding will enhance the effectiveness of the encounter. Remember, clues are an indication that the patient has an issue(s) that is impacting life (and perhaps health) in a significant manner. For the patient this issue, and the emotions it engenders, often dominates his or her life. In the clinical encounter, it can get in the way of the patient's ability to deal with the physical issues that are present, perhaps even rendering the patient incapable of genuinely listening to and interacting with the physician. The patient, seeking relief, will present the clue over and over, deflecting from the medical issue at hand. By hearing and responding, the physician provides the release necessary so the patient can move on. An effective model will be one that incorporates listening and enables the physician to work with the patient in a manner that facilitates openness, directness, and depth.

A final commonly cited barrier

A final commonly cited barrier to the integration of medicine and spirituality is a lack of training. Physicians insist, and rightly so, that they are not trained as theologians or spiritual counselors. They worry that they will attempt to move into the realm of the spiritual with a patient, and it will work! What will they do with such a patient? How will they respond? How can they keep from doing more harm than good? An effective model of integration will not insist that the physician be either a priest or a psychotherapist. It must define an appropriate role for the physician. At Oregon Health and Science University (OHSU) it is believed that the core role of the physician when dealing with spirituality is listening. Thus the core competency taught in the Medicine and Spirituality curriculum is active listening skills. The model in use at this medical school assumes that the physicians should treat the whole person, including the spiritual, mental, and emotional facets of the person. It also assumes that the movement into these realms must begin with the patient and that when moving into the realm of spirituality, the motivation and focus must both be the patient's. OHSU teaches that it is by listening that the physician enables this process and takes on the role of a facilitator or catalyst. Using active listening skills the physician gathers the free information offered by the patient, and uses that information to help the patient express what they want and need to say. The physician does not take control of the conversation or determine the agenda. By providing training in active listening, OHSU enables its graduates to approach the whole person. This is only one example of how appropriate strategies for intervention can be established.

Patient barriers

Earlier we looked at the issue of boundaries primarily from the perspective of the provider. It should be noted that the integration of spirituality in medicine may also create boundary issues for patients. Those who do not consider themselves 'spiritual' may feel uncomfortable by any movement into this realm. This may be, in part, a matter of linguistics, as people have widely varying views about what it means to be spiritual. But this is certainly a significant issue. That is why the kind of training described above is so important. If the approach is truly patient-centered unwanted intrusion can be avoided.

There may also be reasons for even those who consider themselves spiritual to hesitate to move into the realm of the spiritual. Although the research shows that most patients are open to this move,[53] there are barriers. First, many patients may simply prefer spiritual issues to be dealt with within the context of their community of faith. They want spiritual support, but prefer to receive it from their religious leader and their system (through prayer, ritual, etc.). Second, people may be reluctant to examine and confront their deepest issues. They may fear that those issues will be uncomfortable, even shaming. Third, some may actually fear that if they address their spiritual issues the tentative connection they feel to the sacred may be lost. For them their sense of the sacred may be marginal, but helpful. We might liken this mentality to the rock climber who is caught in a difficult and tenuous position and fears to seek a more secure hold for fear of falling.

Questions for reflection

- What are, for you, the major concerns regarding the integration of spirituality and medicine?
- What are the principles for integration that you feel are most critical?
- Explore your own feelings about sharing your spiritual issues with another person. What makes your reluctant to discuss those issues? What motivates you to discuss those issues?

A model for integration

When thinking about the interface of medicine and spirituality it appears that the basic need is for a model of integration that encourages physicians to treat the patient as a whole person, addressing not only physical issues, but also social, emotional, and spiritual issues. This model should provide the physician with the ability to identify patients who are struggling with such issues and the tools for responding to such issues in an appropriate manner. But at the same time this model should take into account the serious issues of time, boundaries, and respect for the deep and complex nature of spiritual and emotional issues.

With these thoughts in mind it is proposed that a sound model for integration will include the following:

1 an understanding of the whole person
2 an appreciation of the essential unity of the person, and how the various facets of personhood affect one another
3 a working concept of spirituality and religiosity, and the impact of these factors on life (and health)
4 active-listening skills and other tools that encourage the patient to share safely and freely about such issues, providing new self-awareness on the part of the patient, and in some cases spiritual relief
5 assessment tools for the identification of spiritual/emotional issues
6 appropriate and effective referral of the patient to a 'spiritual specialist,' one trained to deal with spiritual issues in a longer-term, deeper manner
7 ongoing communication with the patient and their specialist about this aspect of the person's healing process.

Notes

1 Smith NK (trans.) (1958) *Descartes Philosophical Writings*. Random House Inc., Toronto, Canada, p.xi.
2 Smith NK (trans.) (1958) *Descartes Philosophical Writings*. Random House Inc., Toronto, Canada, p.106.
3 Smith NK (trans.) (1958) *Descartes Philosophical Writings*. Random House Inc., Toronto, Canada, p.106.
4 Smith NK (trans.) (1958) *Descartes Philosophical Writings*. Random House Inc., Toronto, Canada, p.xiii.
5 Warhaft S (ed.) (1965) *Francis Bacon, A Selection of His Works, The New Organon*. Odyssey Press, New York, NY, pp.331–92.
6 Stewart M, Brown JB, Weston WW, McWhinney IR, McWilliam C and Freeman TR (1995) *Patient Centered Medicine*. Sage Publications, Thousand Oaks, CA, pp.4–5 (Quoting Faber K *Nosography in Modern Internal Medicine*. (Jean Marting (trans.)). Paul B Hoeber, New York, NY, p.35.)
7 Engel G (1977) The need for a new medical model: a challenge for biomedicine. *Science*. **196**: 129–36; Miller WR (ed.) (1999) *Integrating Spirituality into Treatment*. American Psychological Association, Washington DC, p.3.
8 Pascal B (trans. Trotter WF) (1958) *Pensees*. EP Dutton and Co, New York, NY.
9 Benson H (1996) *Timeless Healing*. A Fireside Book (Simon and Schuster), New York, NY.
10 Gordon JS (1996) *Manifesto for a New Medicine*. Addison Wesley, Reading, MA.
11 Miller WR (ed.) (1999) *Integrating Spirituality into Treatment*. American Psychological Association, Washington DC, pp.6,7.

12   Mandel AJ (1980) Toward a psychobiology of transcendence: God in the brain. In: RJ Davidson and JM Davidson (eds) *The Psychobiology of Consciousness.* Plenum, New York, NY, pp.379–479.

13   Freud S ([1919] 1962) Future of an Illusion. In: J Strachey (ed. and trans.) *Standard Edition of the Complete Psychological Works of Sigmund Freud.* Hogarth Press, London, p.43.

14   Watters W (1992) *Deadly Doctrine: health, illness, and Christian God-talk.* Prometheus, Buffalo, NY, p.12.

15   Ellis A (1980) Psychotherapy and atheistic values: a response to A.E. Bergin's 'Psychotherapy and religious values.' *Journal of Consulting and Clinical Psychology.* **48**: 635–9.

16   Koenig HG, McCullough ME and Larson DB (2001) *Handbook of Religion and Health.* Oxford University Press, Oxford, pp.64–70.

17   Koenig HG, McCullough ME and Larson DB (2001) *Handbook of Religion and Health.* Oxford University Press, Oxford, pp.74–7.

18   Literature search by Oregon Health and Science University faculty in the Department of Family Medicine. Stephen Kliewer, D.Min., Elizabeth Steiner, MD, 1999.

19   Larson DB, Swyers JP and McCullough ME (1997) *Scientific Research on Spirituality and Health: a consensus report.* National Institute for Healthcare Research, Rockville, MD.

20   Koenig HG (1997) *Is Religion Good for Your Health?* Haworth Pastoral Press, New York, NY.

21   Koenig HG, McCullough ME and Larson DB (2001) *Handbook of Religion and Health.* Oxford University Press, Oxford.

22   Larson DB, Swyers JP and McCullough ME (1997) *Scientific Research on Spirituality and Health: a consensus report.* National Institute for Healthcare Research, Rockville, MD.

23   Zinnbauer BJ, Pargament KI, Cole B, Rye MS, Butter EM, Belavich TG *et al.* (1998) Religion and spirituality: unfuzzying the fuzzy. *Journal for the Scientific Study of Religion.* **36**: 549–64.

24   Gopinath N, Chada S, Jain P, Shekhawat S and Tandon R (1995) An epidemiological study of coronary heart disease in different ethnic groups in a Delhi urban population. *Journal of the Association of Physicians of India.* **43**: 30–3.

25   Shang J and Jin S (1996) Determinants of suicide ideation: a comparison of Chinese and American college students. *Adolescence.* **31**(122): 451–67.

26   Daaleman TP and Nease DE Jr (1994) Patient attitudes regarding physician inquiry into spiritual and religious issues. *J Fam Pract.* **39**: 564–8.

27   Gallup G Jr and Lindsay DM (1999) *Surveying the Religious Landscape: trends in US beliefs.* Morehouse, Harrisburg, PA, p.21.

28   Ehman JW, Ott BB and Short TH (1999) Do patients want physicians to inquire about their spiritual or religious beliefs if they become gravely ill? *Arch Intern Med.* **159**: 1803–6.

29   McNichol T (1996) The new faith in medicine. *USA Weekend.* **April 5–7**: 4–5.

30   King DE and Bushwick B (1994) Beliefs and attitudes of hospital inpatients about faith healing and prayer. *J Fam Pract.* **39**: 349–52.

31   Daaleman TP and Frey B (1999) Spiritual and religious beliefs and practices of family physicians: a national survey. *J Fam Pract.* **48**(2): 98–104.

32   Graigie F and Hobbs R III (1999) Spiritual perspectives and practices of family physicians with an expressed interest in spirituality. *Fam Med.* **31**(8): 578–85.

33   Ellis M, Vinson D and Ewigman B (1999) Addressing spiritual concerns with patients: family physicians attitudes and practices. *J Fam Pract.* **48**(2): 105–9.

34   Sloan RP, Bagiella E, VandeCreek L *et al.* (2000) Should physicians prescribe religious activities? *N Engl J Med.* **342**: 1913–16 (Sounding Board).

35   Sloan RP, Bagiella E and Powell T (1999) Religion, spirituality, and medicine. *The Lancet.* **353**: 664–7.

36   Koenig HG, McCullough ME and Larson DB (2001) *Handbook of Religion and Health.* Oxford University Press, Oxford, p.465.

37 Seeman TE, Dubin LF and Seeman M (2003) Religiosity/spirituality and health: a critical review of the evidence for biological pathways. *Am Psychologist.* **58**: 53–63.

38 The talk was given by Stephen Kliewer, D.Min as part of the Principles of Clinical Medicine Course (PCM Session 111). As a result of this encounter the content of the talk was changed.

39 Byrd RC (1988) Positive therapeutic effects of intercessory prayer in a coronary care unit population. *Southern Medical Journal.* **81**: 826–9.

40 Koenig HG (1999) *The Healing Power of Faith: how belief and prayer can help you triumph over disease.* Touchstone Books (Simon & Schuster), New York, NY.

41 Matthews D (1998) *The Faith Factor.* Viking, New York, NY, p.15.

42 Larchet J-C (2002) *The Theology of Illness.* St Vladamir's Seminary Press, Crestwood, NY, p.47.

43 Dostoevsky F (Vintage Books Edition 1955) *The Brothers Karamazov.* Vintage Russian Library, New York, NY.

44 Myss C (1996) *Anatomy of the Spirit.* Three Rivers Press, New York, NY, p.286.

45 Myss C (1996) *Anatomy of the Spirit.* Three Rivers Press, New York, NY, p.199.

46 Myss C (1996) *Anatomy of the Spirit.* Three Rivers Press, New York, NY, p.219.

47 Post SG, Puchalski CM and Larson DB (2000) Physicians and patient spirituality: professional boundaries, competency, and ethics. *Annals of Internal Medicine.* **132**(7): 578–83.

48 Campolo T (1983) *The Power Delusion.* SP Publications (Victor Press), Wheaton, IL, pp.9, 10.

49 Campolo T (1983) *The Power Delusion.* SP Publications (Victor Press), Wheaton, IL, p.11.

50 Campolo T (1983) *The Power Delusion.* SP Publications (Victor Press), Wheaton, IL, p.58.

51 Campolo T (1983) *The Power Delusion.* SP Publications (Victor Press), Wheaton, IL, p.58.

52 Levinson W, Gorawara-Bhat R and Lamb J (2000) A study of patient clues and physician responses in primary care and surgical settings. *JAMA.* **284**(8): 1021–7.

53 Ehman JW, Ott BB and Short TH (1999) Do patients want physicians to inquire about their spiritual or religious beliefs if they become gravely ill? *Arch Intern Med.* **159**(15): 1803–6.

CHAPTER 3

Exploring spirituality

Is anxiety a disease or an addiction? Perhaps it is something of both. Partly, perhaps, because you can't help it, and partly because of some dark reason you choose not to help it, you torment yourself with detailed vision of the worst that can possibly happen. The nagging headache turns out to be a malignant brain tumor.

Friedrich Beuchner, *Whistling in the Dark*

He sat in the chair, his entire body exuding a sense of hopelessness and despair. Shoulders sagging, hands clasped in his lap, head bowed, eyes fixed on a dirty spot on the carpet, his voice was low and flat. He came to the clinic because his life was unraveling. Haltingly he shared a litany of woes. His job was in jeopardy, he felt no sense of intimacy with his wife, and his children treated him with disrespect. 'I'm not surprised my children don't like me,' he shared, 'I don't like myself.' He was drinking heavily and behaving in ways that made him feel like 'a creep.' Finally, he ended his comments by saying, 'I think some of the problem is that I'm just not spiritual.'

Some people picture spirituality as something independent or outside the self. It is something equivalent to a lifestyle choice – one can choose to be spiritual, or not. This leads people to quantify spirituality and talk in terms of being 'more spiritual' or 'less spiritual,' as though it can be measured on a Likert scale. 'Today, on a scale from 1–5, I am a 4, spiritually speaking.' To think about spirituality in this manner is to do it a disservice. We have asserted that all people are inherently spiritual. Each man or woman has a spiritual component that exists and is a part of their essential personhood. It is there, whether acknowledged and nurtured, or denied and ignored. People are physical, social, emotional, and spiritual.

People's struggles to identify their spiritual domain arise for a number of reasons. First there is a failure to understand the nature of spirituality and the way in which the spiritual aspect of our personhood is integrally connected with the totality of the self. Since the spiritual is often difficult to define, people tend to concentrate on the more easily accessible aspects of the self, their bodies, emotions, and social contacts. In some cases the spiritual, because it is integrally related to these other aspects of the self, gets merged with them and loses its own identity. Second, as we have discussed, there is the ongoing confusion between spirituality and religion. Many people, not being involved in religious practices, consider themselves 'not spiritual,' confusing the lack of religiosity with a lack of spirituality. A third key issue is the complexity of spirituality. Spirituality is multidimensional and those unaware of these dimensions may fail to recognize when they are functioning in the realm of the spiritual.

The dimensions of spirituality

There have been many attempts to capture the complexity of spirituality by defining its various dimensions. The taxonomy of dimensions vary, with some including aspects that are primarily religious, some focusing on elements not connected to the religious context, and others including a mix of dimensions, both religious and general. Charles Ndlela suggests six dimensions:[1] His first dimension is *ideological* and involves a person's beliefs or values. The second is *intellectual*, having to do with raw knowledge. The intellectual is differentiated from the ideological because the content being worked with has not been internalized, it has not moved from the brain to the heart (or soul). Some knowledge explored on the intellectual level may not be adopted and made part of one's ideology. The third dimension is the *ritualistic*. On the surface this dimension may appear to be exclusively religious. It is easy to think only in terms of religious rituals that fit clearly into this dimension, such as Christian baptism, Islamic prayers, or the Jewish Seder. However, there are also personal activities that do not fit into the traditional concept of ritual but are very ritualistic. Walking at a certain time each day to think and meditate or going to one specific place to connect with the sacred, and thus creating a 'holy place' can be ritualistic. A fourth dimension is the *experiential*. This is a dimension greatly valued by such religious groups as charismatic Christians and Jewish mystics, but not easily understood by other parts of the religious spectrum. This is the domain of the spiritual experience and has to do with feeling the presence of the divine or sacred, sensing a connection to something greater than one's self. For some it is experiencing the power of the Spirit, the present power of God and the third person of the Christian Trinity. For others it is feeling connected to nature while viewing a dramatic sunset. For some it might even be found in the intimacy of a human relationship. The fifth dimension is the *consequential*. This dimension has to do with the influence of spirituality on everyday activities. When people are moved by the spiritual side of their being and choose to behave in a certain manner because of their beliefs, they are in the dimension of the consequential. This dimension of spirituality gets a lot of attention as it is more concrete than many of the dimensions and can include such diverse behaviors as abstinence, charitable actions, facilitation of social reform, and political involvement. The final dimension for Ndlela is the *supportive*. This is the aspect of spirituality that involves social support or participation in a community and can take many forms. Sometimes it might be overtly religious and involve an institution such as a church or synagogue. At other times the concept of community might be broader and include something as informal as a discussion group that meets at a local coffee house. Community can even include one-on-one supportive relationships.

William Miller and Carl Thoresen distill the spiritual dimensions down to three domains: 'practice, belief and experience.'[2] *Practice* refers to outward actions, specifically to spiritual practices, both individualistic and communal.

> People can be described by the extent to which they engage in spiritual practices such as prayer, fasting, meditation, and contemplation. Also included here would be participation in specifically religious activities such as worship, dance, scriptural study, singing, confession, offerings, and public prayer.[3]

It would be possible to define this domain even more widely to include what Ndlela calls the 'consequential' and include spiritually motivated social behavior such as charitable and social actions. If approached in this manner this domain could even include a lifestyle choice such as a healthy diet. Many people see the body as belonging to God, or being sacred in its own right, and feel compelled to take care of it by eating health food, watching their weight, and abstaining from potentially harmful substances such as alcohol.

The domain of *belief* is quite large and includes the 'existential' issues, questions about life, death, and meaning. What does it mean to be human? What is the nature of personhood? Is there a God, or a spiritual dimension to life? What is the nature of God or the sacred? How does God, or the divine or sacred, relate to humankind? How does humankind connect to the divine? Is there an afterlife, and what is its nature? How should a person live? What is moral? Although not quite as easy to define as the domain of practice, which is the easiest to quantify and measure, this realm is fairly accessible and people can gain entry to it through scriptures and other sacred writings.

The final domain, which is *spiritual experience*, is probably the most difficult to define and measure. This domain involves the actual interaction of the person with the sacred, the person's experience of the divine (in whatever way they define it). What makes this domain difficult is the fact that the interaction occurs in many ways, at many times, and creates a variety of experience.

Ann was the victim of sexual abuse by her father. For years she had struggled to live a normal life. She was angry and alienated, unable to sustain long-term friendships with either men or women. She lived alone, was extremely isolated, and had very poor social skills. Having been raised in an evangelical church, she felt unable to connect with God, who was presented to her almost exclusively as 'Father.' Her unresolved issues with her earthly father left her unable to access God through this image. She wandered from church to church, attempting to 'find God,' but would rarely make it through an entire service of worship. Often, a phrase in a song or reading, or even a comment in a sermon, would anger or confuse her, and she would simply get up and walk out.

One day, while reading a book about Eastern spirituality in a local coffee nook/bookstore, she suddenly dissolved into tears, and then laughter. From that moment forth she was a new person. She smiled frequently, began to be involved with others socially, and found a small group of people with whom she would meet to discuss 'spiritual ideas.' In that moment and place she had what she defined as a spiritual experience and her life was transformed. To this day she cannot explain exactly what happened, or why. All she knows is that it was very real.

Shirley is a woman who has very strong spiritual beliefs. Over the years her faith has been very fluid, and has found expression in a variety of places. While always involved exclusively with the Christian faith, she moved from Mainline Protestantism, where the emphasis is on God as Father and the nurturing creative activity of the divine, to Evangelical Christianity, where the emphasis is on God the Son (Jesus) and on the judging and saving acts of God, to Pentecostalism, where the focus is on the Spirit and the present power of God. Now she has a very personalized form of Christian faith, heavily focused on the Spirit. One day while shopping with a friend in a very busy store she came upon a register that was just being opened. All around were lines several persons long. She was able to move directly to the counter. Shirley exclaimed 'Oh a blessing!' For her this was a spiritual experience.

What is a spiritual experience? These two profiles illustrate that a spiritual experiences are highly personal and may vary significantly from person to person. Some people may see absolutely nothing as a spiritual experience, while for others spiritual experiences are dramatic and spectacular, moments when the normal patterns of the world are broken. For yet others spiritual experience involves the everyday, perhaps even the routine. How do we define what is spiritual and what is not? It is clear that two people can have essentially the same experience, but affix different meaning to the event. It may not be possible to come up with a satisfactory objective definition. Perhaps it is best just to remember that spirituality is more than a set of beliefs, or a set of behaviors, but is also something we 'experience.'

It really doesn't matter how many domains one identifies, or even how one defines those domains. What is important is that we understand and respect the complexity of spirituality as we explore our spirituality, or that of another. What is the content of all the domains for this unique person? What do they believe? How have they experienced the sacred? How does their spirituality translate into practice?

In exploring a person's unique spirituality there are a number of ways we can use the domains to gain a clearer understanding of a person's spiritual dynamics. First there is the actual content of the domains. For the purposes of discussion let us use Miller and Thoresen's three domains, belief, practice, and experience. What, for example, is the content of the belief domain? What is the nature of the divine? Is the divine generous or demanding? Does God interact with human kind? If so, how? Does the sacred or divine intervene in human history, or is it a more passive power?

It is important at this point to note that some people have 'pathological beliefs,' ones that are inherently unhealthy... This is not a matter of theological differences, but relates to thoughts that would generally be accepted as inappropriate. One example might be the person who believes God, or whatever power they relate to, is calling him to kill himself or another person. A pathological belief might also be one that is in direct contradiction of the 'facts,' such a belief that one could jump off a tall building and not be harmed.

There are also beliefs that might be classified as 'troublesome,' at least from a health and spirituality perspective. A belief that God 'causes' illness as a way of punishing or teaching people might be one example. This is certainly a matter of theological debate, with some religious systems clearly believing that God is in control of and causes everything, including illness. It is clear what kind of difficulty this might create for a person who is ill. If they are ill, they must have done something bad. If they have done something bad, they deserve to be ill. If they deserve to be ill...? This mentality is pictured in a humorous way in the Peanuts cartoon in Figure 3.1.

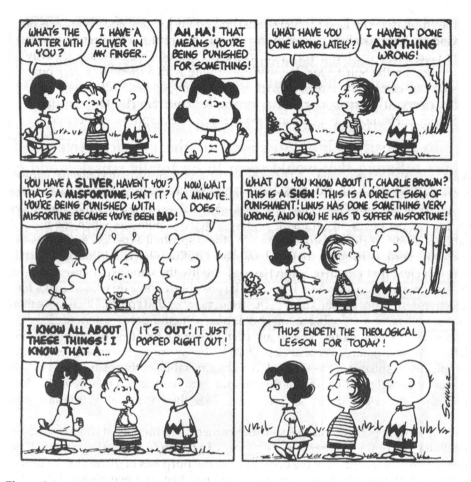

Figure 3.1

Peanuts © United Feature Syndicate, Inc.

Not only must we look at the content of the domains, but we must also explore the way the domains relate to one another. Do these domains complement one another, or conflict with one another? Using Miller or Thoresen's domains, do a person's beliefs 'line up' with his experience of spirituality? Using Ndlela's domains, is a person's consequential domain in alignment with their belief domain? Are her stated values reflected in the way she lives? In other words, is their congruency between the domains? In particular, is there consistency between the 'head and heart' aspects of one's spirituality and one's life? Ideally all domains are congruent. However, it is possible for there to be a state of incongruence between the spiritual domains. A person may, for example, be engaged in a lifestyle that violates some of the values present in the domain of belief. In this case the practice domain (or consequential) is not congruent with the belief domain. If there is incongruence there may be a degree of spiritual discomfort.

What is most important is what happens when the content of the domains and their relationship to one another interface with significant 'outside' factors. Life happens! How does a person apply their spirituality to life events such as death, illness, and failure. What is their 'spiritual thinking' as they move through daily life? For our purposes we are defining 'spiritual thinking' as that which is produced by both the content of a person's domains and the way those domains relate to one another.

In some cases a person's spiritual thinking will clearly be unhelpful. People will see illness as a punishment, or be without hope of healing. They will see themselves as isolated and cut off from the sacred. How has the content of their spiritual domains and/or the way those domains related to one another contributed to these thoughts? The factor that creates spiritual tension may be the content of one particular domain. As we have noted, there are pathological beliefs that by their very nature create distress. In other cases the tension may occur because one domain does not align with another. A person may believe that they should always act in a loving manner, but be in a significant conflict with another person.

Table 3.1 illustrates a number of possible scenarios. The content of the domains varies from person to person, as does the degree of congruity. The table shows how these variations might create diverse spiritual thoughts, and how those thoughts might support or hinder healing.

What is useful about this approach to spirituality is that it provides a framework for analyzing the spiritual thoughts being presented by patients. The 'domain model' respects the complexity of spirituality. It focuses not only on belief, but also on outward practices and personal experiences. It can help us explore facets of spirituality that might otherwise be neglected. All too often our focus is unbalanced, concentrating on one aspect or another. Generally we tend to place our focus on that aspect of spirituality that is most important, or at times, most troubling to us. By looking carefully at all the domains, and at the way they relate to one another, no aspect of spirituality is neglected. The result is that we can often gain great understanding about why people think about their illness the way they do. We can get a glimpse into the genesis of both the negative and positive spiritual thoughts that so affect the process of healing.

The strength of this approach is also its weakness. To explore the concept of healthy spirituality from the perspective of spiritual domains is to focus on a model that is highly 'content' oriented. Because of the nature of spiritual content, difficult issues emerge. Who decides which beliefs are pathological or troubling and which are healthy? The domain of belief (Miller/Thoresen) can have wildly different content, depending on the faith system involved and the culture in which the person is immersed. Christians, for example, often judge any other belief system to be false. Others have a more inclusive perspective, but still may have beliefs that conflict with those of other systems. Since beliefs significantly influence practice (Miller/Thoresen), ritual (Ndlela), and experience (Miller/Thoresen), there is a great deal of diversity within those two domains as well. Indeed, it is impossible to think of a domain in which there is not a diversity of content. This can create real issues when people with differing spiritual frameworks interact.

David was a 48-year-old man who was diagnosed with pancreatic cancer. Upon hearing of this diagnosis his immediate response was to say, 'I should have known.' His physician was rather curious about this response, which seemed a bit unusual. Upon talking to David the physician learned that David believed God was punishing him for marital infidelity. David's church believed that God was in control of absolutely everything, and that nothing,

Continued on p. 54

Table 3.1 Domain-focused case scenarios

Domain	Congruence present / Content not problematic	Incongruence present / Content not problematic	Incongruence present / Content problematic	Congruence present / Content problematic (beliefs conflict with life event)
		Dynamic		
Beliefs	God is loving and forgiving. The world is fallen, and bad things happen, but God does not cause evil. God expects me to act in love toward others. God expects me to honor my promises. God expects me to live an ethical life (obey the Ten Commandments).	God is loving and forgiving. The world is fallen, and bad things happen, but God does not cause evil. God expects me to act in love toward others. God expects me to honor my promises. God expects me to live an ethical life (obey the Ten Commandments).	God is a stern and demands obedience. The world is fallen, and bad things happen because of sin. God is in control of everything. God expects me to act in love toward others. God expects me to honor my promises. God expects me to live an ethical life (obey the Ten Commandments).	God is loving and forgiving. The world is fallen, and bad things happen. God expects me to act in love toward others. God expects me to honor my promises. God expects me to live an ethical life (obey the Ten Commandments). God is in control of everything.
Practice	Worship is important. It is good to study the Bible, pray, and have other spiritual practices. It is important to participate in the church's rituals, such as communion.	Worship is important. It is good to study the Bible, pray, and have other spiritual practices. It is important to participate in the church's rituals, such as communion.	Worship is central to the spiritual life and participation in a church is mandatory for one to be 'in grace.' One is 'in' or 'out.' The church is the 'keeper' of grace. It is good to study the Bible, pray, and have other spiritual practices.	It is important to practice spiritual disciplines. The Bible is the only 'voice' for God. The sacraments of the church are a necessary part of the spiritual life.
Experience	I was born in the church and God has always been a part of my life. God's presence is real, but my experience of God is not intense.	I was born in the church and God has always been a part of my life. God's presence is real, but my experience of God is not intense.	I have chosen to be a part of the church, and am only at peace with God when I am in fellowship and am following God's rules rigorously. If I obey God I will be blessed, if I disobey I will be judged.	I have had a powerful religious experience and have become 'saved'.

continued

Table 3.1 Continued

Impact	Healthy	Unhealthy	Healthy	Unhealthy
Life situation	I am a faithful member of a church. I have a serious illness. I have lived a good life.	I am a faithful member of a church. I have a serious illness. I have embezzled funds.	I am a member of a church. I have a serious illness. I have embezzled funds.	I am a member of God's church. I live a good life. I have a serious illness.
Spiritual thoughts	My illness is a negative thing and is related to living in a 'fallen' world. God loves me. God will work with me to create healing, if not cure. I will use my community of faith and my spiritual practices to help me cope.	I have things in my life that need work. My illness is a negative thing but has nothing to do with my behavior. God loves me and will work with me to create healing in all areas of my life. I will use my community of faith and my spiritual practices to cope with my illness and straighten out my life.	I have things in my life that need work. My illness is due to my behavior. God is punishing me through my illness. My church will disown me if they find out about my behavior. I will be shunned. I deserve to be ill. I don't deserve to get well.	I think I have been a good person, but I am ill. Only people who have sinned get ill! What have I done to deserve this? Why has God abandoned me? I am angry at God! I am in sin for feeling angry!
Outcomes	Healthy spiritual thoughts that support and encourage and facilitate healing.	Healthy spiritual thoughts that facilitate change, growth, and healing.	Unhealthy spiritual thoughts that hinder healing and hope.	Unhealthy spiritual thoughts that hinder healing.

even illness, occurred without God's initiation. David, who was feeling extremely guilty because of his behavior, and having a theological perspective that invoked a simplistic cause and effect formula, saw the meaning of his illness as punishment. While the physician saw David's spirituality as unhealthy, David and his pastor did not. They were totally comfortable framing David's illness in the manner. Indeed it would have been far more damaging, from their perspective, to 'ignore' God's message than it was to understand and accept the illness as God's 'refining and purifying' action.

Other problems can emerge when the focus of spiritual exploration becomes the content. There can be an intellectualization of spirituality that allows for compartmentalization. One can talk about the content of faith for a long time without ever getting to the level of the heart, or without ever exploring how the spirituality integrates with the rest of life. If not careful, the domain model may direct us further into the realm of religion, with its established scriptures (beliefs), rituals (practices), and communities (in which one 'experiences' the divine).

However, in spite of its weaknesses the domain model remains an excellent tool for exploring one's own spirituality. It can also provide great insight into the spirituality of others. Again the task is twofold. First, to define for oneself the domains of spirituality (pick a set that make sense to you personally), and then explore the content of those domains. Second, to think about the relationships of the various domains to one another, and to the way they impact your own personal reality.

For reflection

- Think about your own spirituality.
- What are some of the key concepts of values that comprise your spiritual beliefs?
- What are, for you, the most important spiritual practices?
- Describe your most intense experience of God.
- Think about how you 'normally' experience the sacred or divine (however you define it).
- Is your 'reality' consistent with your spiritual domains?
- How do you 'value' or think about illness? What is your spiritual thinking?

Spirituality as journey

Another way to approach personal spirituality is to explore it from the perspective of spiritual imagery. One of the most common spiritual images is that of quest. The concept of quest or journey is found extensively throughout spiritual literature and involves a search for the sacred or the divine (personified or not), or a search for meaning, understanding, or wholeness. There have been many versions of the journey image or model, including Bunyan's *Pilgrim's Progress*, CS Lewis' *Voyage of the Dawn Treader*, various Greek Myths, and the journeys of Buddha.

The major focal point in the journey or quest image is the process. The quest presents spirituality as an ongoing process where one incorporates spiritual experience and finds spiritual transformation. This journey mentality is reflected in Joseph Campbell's book *The Hero with a Thousand Faces*.[4] In this book Campbell focuses on the hero who is, essentially, a person who wants to maximize existence, a person seeking spiritual growth. According to Campbell's story the essential trait of a 'hero in the making' is restlessness or inner strife. Growth begins when a person is not at ease with his/her immediate environment and circumstances. The quest begins when unease gnaws at the heart, prompting the person to question the very nature of existence. It is this divine discomfort that mobilizes the person, moves them to undertake the journey. Campbell divides the journey into five distinct phases.

1 The call to adventure.
2 Crossing of the threshold (entering the unknown).
3 Trials and tribulations of the journey.
4 Attainment of enlightenment.
5 Return of the hero.

The Buddha's journey to spiritual awakening or 'Nirvana,' as it is popularly called, perfectly mirrors the above-mentioned progressive development of a hero.

In essence, the 'journey' model leads to what has been called a 'process definition' of spirituality.[5] A process definition pays attention to the spiritual journey that is taking place, to the spiritual transformation that occurs, rather than to the mechanisms or content involved.[6] With a process definition, therefore, the evaluation of a person's spirituality is focused on what is happening to or within the person. Is this person becoming more open? Is he discovering new meanings? Is she finding a meaning and purpose in life?

This is far different than the domain model that focuses on content and thus involves the contextualization of the process. Contextualization involves identification with a specific power, such as Yahweh, Allah, Higher Power, God, or Mother Earth. It encourages alliance with specific faith systems, such as Judaism, Buddhism, Hinduism, Christianity, or Islam. With contextualization there is a focus on specific bodies of knowledge, such as the Torah, the Bible, the Koran, or other religious writings, and a resultant accent on specific doctrines. There is also an emphasis on specific activities and rituals, such as baptism, communion, the Seder, a pilgrimage to Mecca, or meditation. When we contextualize we move ourselves toward the realm of religion rather than spirituality.

Change or growth is central to the journey model. The person is on a journey where, with the help of whatever context they have chosen, they find the capacity to take what happens in their lives, process that event and the feelings it engenders, and create meaning, perhaps new meaning. The critical result is that one moves beyond where one was, to a place that is somehow higher, broader, and more inclusive. One moves beyond seeing illness, for example, as a punishment, to seeing it as a part of life. This allows one to respond to the illness differently.

In this model one essentially must walk a narrow path balancing what the author called openness and groundedness.[7] Openness involves being open to the sacred, to spiritual experiences. Groundedness involves being attentive to outer reality. If one becomes unbalanced and moves too far to one side or the other, growth stops and spiritual wellness is jeopardized. If one becomes too 'grounded' for example, one becomes spiritually repressed, and is unable to be open to the spiritual dimension. If one becomes too open, one may experience a spiritual emergency. The ability to integrate one's spirituality into the rest of life can be lost. Spirituality actually becomes a detriment to work, relationships, or even the self as one becomes disconnected with reality.[8] Following is an example of a person who struggled with spiritual repression.

Howard is a 75-year-old man who developed slowly progressive Parkinson's disease about five years ago. Previously an active church member, he had enjoyed remarkably good health throughout his life until the time of his diagnosis. Soon after learning of his illness, he actively learned everything he could about the disease. He visited multiple physicians and insisted on being referred to the best academic health center in his area to get state-of-the-art care. Based on advice from his many physicians, he radically changed his diet and his daily activities. He used several medications and dietary supplements and kept careful records of his care plan. As the condition worsened, Howard felt that he was failing to respond because he had not yet found the best medical plan. He became obsessed with his healthcare and, as his ability to walk and talk became affected, withdrew from social interactions, including his church. Approaching the end of his life, he was lonely and depressed and he felt abandoned by his community of faith.

On the opposite end of the spectrum is the person who lives in the realm of spiritual emergency.

Mary and Joshua were married and had two children, aged 5 and 8. Mary was devoutly religious and attended church twice each week, but Joshua found organized religion to be hypocritical and boring. While Mary went to church, Joshua would read books of philosophy and poetry. He supported Mary's desire to raise their children in the church. Soon after his fifth birthday, their son Eric died in a drowning accident in a neighbor's swimming pool. The family was devastated by the loss. Mary turned to her faith and received support from other church members, but Joshua felt that Eric's death proved that God either did not exist or did not care about his family. His opposition to religion became more strident, and Mary responded by viewing his lack of faith as a spiritual explanation for Eric's death. Like many families after the death of a child, they drew apart and ultimately separated, with Joshua moving out and beginning to drink heavily.

To move back more directly to the image of journey, when one is too grounded one is essentially 'stuck.' Perhaps the image of the car sunk up to the axles in mud is an appropriate picture. When one is too open, one is lost, wandering around in the wilderness with no clear point of reference. Although most of us will be 'stuck' or 'lost' at some point, the goal is to be moving, on the way toward a place, a goal, a state, or even a person. We can be seeking Nirvana, looking for the Promised Land, trying to 'find God,' or merely striving for inner peace. It should be noted that while many embrace the concept of journey as a meaningful image of the spiritual life, theologically it may not be the most defensible model for Christians. In Christianity, the story is more about God seeking human kind than it is about human kind seeking God. Faith is more about being 'found' by a God who seeks to rebuild a relationship with the created than it is about the person 'finding' the divine. This may lead some to use an alternative image, that of relationship.

For reflection

Illustrate your own spiritual journey. Use whatever method works best for you. Draw your 'path' on a large piece of paper. Illustrate key moments or changes of direction. Write out a spiritual itinerary. Start with the past, and move on into the future. Develop a 'scrapbook.' Use photos or drawings to illustrate your spiritual journey. What have been the key moments in your journey? How have those moments affected you? Changed your direction, your behavior, your thinking? What are some key spiritual values or thoughts that are the result of your journey?

How will those thoughts affect you as you move forward in life?

Spirituality as relationship

Some people, rather than seeing spirituality as a process, tend to see it from a relational perspective. The relational image focuses on the concept of a transforming connection or relationship with something or someone greater than one's self. The connection can be with a reality outside the self, or perhaps one within. This model focuses less on the development or movement of the spiritual self, and more on a sense of connectedness to someone or something greater than the self. This model is very common among people belonging to a faith system that has a divine being, such as Christianity, Judaism, or Islam. However, it is important to note that the model can also be used by people whose spirituality is rooted in nature, or in a loosely defined sense of the sacred or divine. The key is seeing the 'relationship' or sense of 'connectedness' as the heart of spiritual wellness. As one is connected in an empowering and transforming way to what one person calls 'the beyond,'[9] one is capable of being connected to the world, to others, and even to the self in a positive and transforming way.

This model in its most appropriate forms does not assume a relationship that is always comfortable, peaceful, and upbeat. It is, after all, a relationship. So it is natural that there be moments when the relationship is in stress or when the sense of connection falters. What matters most is that the relationship or connection is constantly being nurtured, renegotiated, and redefined. It is alright for the relationship to go through a moment of turmoil as long as the issues are addressed in a real manner and the relationship moves forward, or the connection is redefined or re-energized. With this model, spiritual well-being is lost when relational turmoil occurs, but is not addressed. A person becomes spiritually unhealthy when steps are not taken to restore a connection that is threatened, weakened, or even severed.

A study was once done of people who had dropped out of their Christian communities of faith.[10] The study revealed that people go through a number of stages in their relationships both with the divine (God) and with the community of faith that provides them with a context for that relationship (the Church). Essentially the relationship begins with a period of information gathering and expectation setting. During this 'getting to know you' period the person gathers information about God (or whatever someone or something greater than themselves that is the focus of the relationship) and develops a set of expectations about the relationship. It is what might be called 'spiritual dating.' What is the character or nature of this one, this force, to whom I might become connected? What can I expect to receive from this relationship? What will be expected of me in this relationship? What are the benefits? What are the negatives, the dangers? So in the initial stage the parties in the relationship develop the rules for relating to one another, and the expectations are defined.

If it seems appropriate, a choice is then made to actually make a commitment to the other. One consciously, perhaps formally, enters into the relationship. Once the relationship is entered there is normally a period of productivity and stability. The 'other' appears to fit the definition that was developed during the time of information gathering. The expectations that were established seem to be valid and appropriate. The relationship works and is positive and dynamic. The following cognitive map shows this process of relational development.

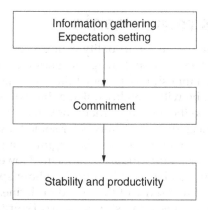

Figure 3.2

What the study also discovered was that at certain times almost everyone's relationship with the divine went through times of disruption.[11] The disruption can be generated by a number of sources. Jobs, the economy, significant relationships, illness, low self-esteem, a community of faith, even a person's belief system; all might trigger the relational crisis. What occurs is that in some way the expectations developed for the relationship are violated. Something happens that was unexpected or unwanted, and the result is discomfort, with the state of stability and productivity being disrupted.

The movement from stability to disruption can vary in terms of time and intensity depending upon the nature of the violation. Violations can be painful, or merely confusing. They can be minor, or significant. At times a single breach might be so powerful that it causes profound disruption. Sometimes the infringements are small and easily ignored, but the impact builds and multiplies until finally a critical mass is reached that causes spiritual turmoil. According to John Savage the product of this unresolved turmoil is anxiety. Anxiety is 'the effect which is produced by an arousal period of short or long duration when persons feel they are knocked off their equilibrium (emotional, psychical, or rational balance).'[12] In other words, a point is reached where there is no security, no confidence in one's belief system, no sense that one knows what to expect.

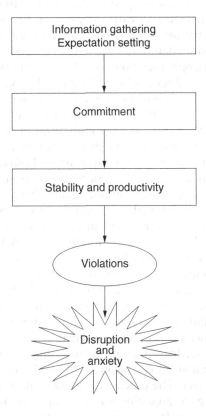

Figure 3.3

There are, according to Savage, different kinds of anxiety. *Real anxiety* is that which is based in fact. A person who has an illness that is life threatening has 'real' anxiety. There is *neurotic anxiety*, which is not based in fact, but is illusory in nature. A person who is constantly in fear and believes they have a terminal or serious illness, when in fact there are no symptoms or facts to support this belief, is suffering from this kind of anxiety. Someone who has the perception that a person (or persons) doesn't like them, when there is no basis for that belief is experiencing neurotic anxiety. There is also *moral anxiety*. This is anxiety based upon a belief, a sense of awareness that one has violated the rules, or perhaps been unfaithful to the relationship. A Christian, for example, who has violated one of the Ten Commandments might well suffer from moral anxiety. Finally there is *existential anxiety*. This is the kind of anxiety that comes as one struggles with the great existential questions. 'Does my life have a purpose?' 'Have I accomplished anything meaningful?' 'What will happen to me when I die?' When a person is in spiritual crisis one or perhaps several of these types of anxiety are likely to be found.

The problem, as noted earlier, is not the anxiety itself but what occurs when the anxiety is not dealt with appropriately. A disruption of the relationship results in a weakening or a severance of the relational connection with the sacred. This disruption can look very different depending upon the person. Some people, for example, focus outward and place the burden of the disruption on the other party in the relationship. For example, some people get angry with God. Why did he/she allow this to happen? Others turn inward and place the burden of the disruption on themselves. They get angry, but the anger is directed at the self. 'How could I have been so stupid!? I have sinned and no longer deserve God's love.'

Savage suggests that people thus take one of two paths away from the relationship. They either see the problem as being God or whatever power or entity they feel connected to (I'm OK, you're not OK), or they see the problem as being themselves (I'm not OK, you're OK). In the first case they often push others away in anger, isolating themselves from God, their faith community, even other people. In the other case they see themselves as being hopeless, unlovable, of no value to God or others, and turn inward and become withdrawn. In both cases the person who is in spiritual crisis 'seals off' and becomes closed to resolution and change. In the case of those who focus outward, the seal-off often looks like an abrupt termination of the relationship. There is a relational explosion, and a clear sense of separation. In some cases this separation is permanent. In other cases it is temporary and the relationship is re-established, but often without any work being done to prevent future issues. So the reinvestment into the relationship is premature and unexamined In the case of those who focus inward, the separation may be subtler. The person may simply become less active in their community of faith, or stop other personal spiritual practices. There may never have been a clear 'separation' from God, but instead the relationship enters into a state of 'ennui.' There is no vitality, no growth, no movement, just an uncomfortable co-existence.

It is possible, of course, to repair the relationship, even in cases where the violation has been major and the disruption extreme. It involves going back to the beginning and starting over. The process of repairs entails gathering more information, adding, rejecting, or adjusting – redefining expectations, and creating a more functional relationship. In actuality, as with any relationship, it is a never-ending process and an ever-evolving relationship.

For reflection

- Can you think about the sacred in terms of someone or something to be 'related' to?
- How would you describe the nature of that relationship?
- How is your sense of 'connectedness' with the sacred (close, distant, non-existent)?
- When do you feel closest?
- When do you feel most distant?
- Are there any specific issues that are problematic in terms of your relationship?
- What would it take to 'renegotiate' around those issues?

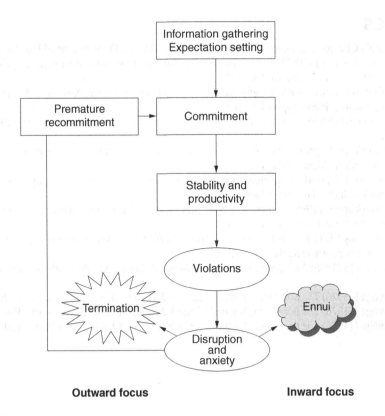

Figure 3.4

Application

Any attempt to address spirituality in the context of healthcare should involve an exploration and understanding of personal spirituality. In the therapeutic relationship, the healthcare professional and the patient must both have at least some rudimentary knowledge of their own spiritual framework and spiritual health. The care providers must understand their own spirituality, since that spirituality is likely to impact beliefs, values and expectations, and the way they interact with the patient. The patients must understand their spirituality, and specifically their spiritual thinking, in order to understand the way their spiritual condition either enables or hinders the process of healing. Spirituality, which is a powerful aspect of the self, does have an impact on illness and its treatment, but it can only be of use if it is explored and understood.

Notes

1   Ndlela Charles J, MD, MPH, University of California, Department of Psychiatry.
2   Miller WR (ed.) (1999) *Integrating Spirituality into Treatment*. American Psychological Association, Washington DC, p.7.
3   Miller WR (ed.) (1999) *Integrating Spirituality into Treatment*. American Psychological Association, Washington DC, p.7.
4   Campbell J (1949) *The Hero with a Thousand Faces*. Princeton University Press, Princeton, NJ.
5   Hinterkopf E (1998) *Integrating Spirituality into Counseling*. American Counseling Association, Alexandria, VA.
6   Gendlin ET (1961) Experiencing: a variable in the process of therapeutic change. *American Journal of Psychotherapy*. **15**: 233–45.
7   Hinterkopf E (1998) *Integrating Spirituality into Counseling*. American Counseling Association, Alexandria, VA, p.3.
8   Hinterkopf E (1998) *Integrating Spirituality into Counseling*. American Counseling Association, Alexandria, VA, p.3–4.
9   Gordon JS (1996) *Manifesto for a New Medicine*. Addison-Wesley Publishing Co, Reading, MA.
10 Savage J (1976) *The Bored and Apathetic Church Member*. LEAD Consultants, Pitford, NY.
11 Savage J (1976) *The Bored and Apathetic Church Member*. LEAD Consultants, Pitford, NY.
12 Savage J (1976) *The Bored and Apathetic Church Member*. LEAD Consultants, Pitford, NY.

CHAPTER 4

The impact of spirituality

Disease is the will speaking through the body, a language for dramatizing the mental: a form of self-expression.

Susan Sontag, *Illness as Metaphor*

A sense of dis-ease

Dr Daniel Fisher MD, PhD, the Executive Director of the National Empowerment Center, is a proponent of what is called the 'recovery' model of mental healthcare. The recovery model seeks to help people with mental illness develop a sense that life can and will go on and is worth living. In a talk given in 2004 to mental health professionals in Oregon, Dr Fisher noted that most people with mental illness have a common ailment, 'despair about life.' 'Being,' he said, 'people with a lack of purpose, meaning, or sense of self, people with mental illness or addiction issues are vulnerable to coping strategies such as another reality or substance use.'[1]

His comments reflect powerfully what can happen when a spiritual life is not healthy. It is all too possible for a person, no matter how well intentioned, to end up in a spiritual emergency. Such situations occur when spiritual thinking about the sacred, illness, health, even life becomes a barrier to growth and healing. With the spiritual journey or process model, one can become uncentered, and be either repressed or ungrounded. Using the journey image more directly, they become stuck, unable to move, or lost, totally out of touch with reality. With the relationship model the moment always comes (it is normal and predicable) when people experience a disruption in the relationship with their personal source of life and meaning. In these moments people experience what Fisher calls despair and Savage calls anxiety. One senses that life has fallen apart and wonders whether life is worth living. It is a moment when personhood, including spirituality, is shaken, and one is in a state of dis-ease.[2]

In his book *The Bored and Apathetic Church Member*, Savage defines the state of dis-ease, which he calls anxiety, in this manner. 'Anxiety is the affect (feeling) which is produced by an arousal period of short or long duration when persons feel they are knocked off their equilibrium (emotional, psychical, or rational balance).'[3] Anxiety then is a consciousness that things are not right. To return to the models of spirituality, it is connected with incongruence, with an awareness of relational disruption, and with a sense of being out of balance. It may, as has been noted by Savage, take a variety of forms: real, neurotic, moral, and existential. Engles supports a similar range of forms in his book *Psychological Development in Health and*

Disease, noting that anxiety 'may be realistic to varying degrees or totally unrealistic (phobias or delusions).'[4]

Whatever the cause, real or delusional, anxiety is often extremely uncomfortable. According to Engles it 'may range from vague feelings of uneasiness, restlessness and foreboding to specifically identified fears.'[5] Perhaps the power of spiritual anxiety or dis-ease is related to the fact that it is often connected to the great existential issues such as meaning and purpose in life, or the nature and meaning of death. Because of its connection to the existential, many theologians and philosophers, most of whom tie the state of anxiety to spiritual crisis, have addressed the theme of anxiety. It is also important to note that these great thinkers often relate spiritual crisis (and thus anxiety) to loss, either the loss of meaning and purpose or the loss of physical existence. This was a connection made frequently by Paul Tillich, the profound theologian who wrote around the middle of the last century. He wrote:

> The first assertion about the nature of anxiety is this: anxiety is the state in which a being is aware of possible nonbeing.[6]
> Man is not only finite, as is every creature; he is also aware of his finitude. And this awareness is anxiety ... Man experiences the anxiety of losing himself by not actualizing himself and his potentialities[7] (so it is the awareness, again of nonbeing, both physical and otherwise).

According to Tillich, anxiety is created when one is confronted with the awareness, or at least the possibility, of non-being, both physical and spiritual. This sense of non-being is often the result of being unhealthy spiritually – of being lost, disconnected, or incongruent.

Martin Heidegger also believed that an unhealthy spirituality drives people toward a focus on loss and vulnerability. He understood anxiety as an affective disposition that expresses the individual's relatedness to a world that has lost its meaning. It relates to a person's reluctance to accept the actuality and inevitability of their own death.[8]

Over the past quarter century, medicine has tended to focus on biologic aspects of anxiety. Anxiety has been defined as a symptom of mental illness and its biologic causes have been tied by medical research to imbalances in certain neurotransmitters in the central nervous system. This research has resulted in a growing number of medications that reduce or even eliminate the physical manifestations of anxiety. In effect, physicians have at their disposal medications that can reduce or eliminate anxiety without ever addressing its emotional or spiritual dimensions. From a medical point of view, anxiety as a symptom can result from use of stimulant medications, as a symptom of depression or a number of so-called anxiety disorders, or can even reflect disease in other body systems, such as thyroid disease. The 'medicalization' of anxiety is one of the best examples of medicine's profound bias toward physical explanations of patient's experiences at the expense of broader issues in other domains.

Not all authors see anxiety as inherently negative. According to Soren Kierkegaard, the existentialist, anxiety is the painful dizziness that occurs when one comes face to face with the 'abyss' of possibility. It is a danger (if not responded to properly), but also a prod to action, something that leads to creativity.[9] Thus for Kierkegaard, anxiety is not necessarily something that leads to despair, and it is certainly not 'terminal.' It is instead a warning signal, a sign that something is not right in the spiritual realm. It is not inherently a step toward hopelessness, but instead can be a step toward action and, more importantly, hope. This is the essential purpose of this chapter. Why is it critical to explore our spirituality? Why play with these various models in order to come to a deeper understanding of our spiritual health? Because spiritual distress (anxiety) can be both a danger and an opportunity.

The dark side of spirituality
Hopelessness/helplessness

While anxiety may be an uncomfortable and frightening emotional state, its true danger lies in how it impacts those people suffering from spiritual distress. Spiritual anxiety expresses itself in a plethora of ways that can be barriers to healing and wholeness. One of the major byproducts of anxiety is helplessness. Savage, who sees this as a major impact of spiritual distress, notes that, 'helplessness is the affect felt when an individual perceives there is no help from outside of the self. One gives up on any stimuli which might extricate one from a given problem.'[10] It is easy to see how a person who feels disconnected from the sacred or a person who feels lost spiritually might develop this sense of helplessness, a debilitating belief that life will not be worth living because of factors over which they have no control. Not only is there a sense that outside forces are destroying them, there is the companion sense that there is no external resource, such as God or wisdom, to provide them with the ability to respond to the onslaught. Thus people with cancer might well find helplessness both in the cancer, over which they appear to have no control, and in the fact that God doesn't seem to care or choose to act on their behalf.

Mr B is an 84-year-old retired postal worker. He has lived alone since the death of his wife three years ago. Although he has three adult children who live close by, he sees them rarely and spends most of his time watching television. Over the past several years, his health has deteriorated and he takes medication to control Type 2 diabetes. He was diagnosed with Parkinson's disease about a year ago and has experienced functional decline as a result of worsening tremor and weakness.

A crisis occurs when his family finds him on the floor of his house, in poor hygiene without having eaten for a two- to three-day period and he is hospitalized. Mr B does not communicate well with his physicians. He is fearful of his growing loss of independence and feels alone, even though his children are attentive and supportive. He feels no control over his circumstances. Progress in his care begins when a family conference is held allowing him to express his sense of helplessness. His care team and family succeed in giving him a series of choices for his care. After a two-month rehabilitation stay in a nursing home, he chooses to return to his home with assistance from a home nursing agency. He enters hospice care with a plan to spend the last months or years of his life as independently as his condition will allow.

A similar consequence of unresolved spiritual distress is hopelessness. According to Savage, 'hopelessness is the feeling there is no resource inside of the self to solve the problem.'[11] Another author, while describing the spiritual crisis he experienced due to a personal tragedy, describes the hopelessness in this manner:

> In this frame of mind 'everything looks utterly hopeless ... He curses the day he was born and even the night he was conceived and makes it clear that if he could die immediately it would suit him fine.' Meaning totally collapses for him.[12]

One major difference between helplessness and hopelessness is the point of focus. Helplessness is focused outward, while hopelessness is focused inward. With hopelessness, 'I' am unable to deal with life, unable to make the right choices, or perform the right actions. This response may well be connected to shame. There is a fundamental defect in the person that makes resolution of the issue impossible. 'I cannot deal with my behavior because I am bad. Even if God, or some other power were available to help, he/she/it would not, because I am unworthy of such an effort.'

Mr R is a 52-year-old professional struggling with obesity, high blood pressure, and depression. His family physician would like to help him with his weight issue, which is clearly contributing to his hypertension and is probably a factor in his depression. However, Mr R is very uncooperative and seems totally unmotivated. In conversations with his physician he has offered clues that suggest that he sees himself as a 'failure.' He appears to view his weight problem and many other issues as unavoidable. 'It's just the way I am.' 'No matter what I try, it doesn't work.' When asked if he has family or friends who might support him in his efforts he responds, 'Who would ever care for me?' Indeed, his tendency to self-depreciate and focus on his perceived lack of ability is very frustrating for his physician, who at times feels very impatient with Mr R. It is probable that Mr R's lack of action with respect to his life issues, including his physical and relational problems, are rooted in his perception of himself as inherently flawed, and thus as a 'hopeless' case. There are clues in his stories that this sense of hopelessness may have begun after he was involved in 'immoral' behavior that occurred many years earlier. When his 'sin' was exposed, the church he attended at the time publicly announced his error, forced him to make a public apology, and, essentially, drove him away from active participation in the congregation.

There are many possible therapeutic consequences to the presence of helplessness and hopelessness. One potential behavioral outcome is rigidity. Feeling incapable or hopeless, people can become frozen, incapable of moving forward on the journey, unable to reach out relationally to the divine. Their spiritual thinking tells them that whatever action they take, it is bound to be wrong and so they give up. Perhaps they could try to live life fully and joyfully, but why? One author describes what happens when women respond to aging and the inexorable movement toward mortality with helplessness. Feeling totally helpless, unable to stop a process they see as negative, they essentially stop living. 'Paradoxically this course, instead of prolonging life, by keeping our bodies rigid, trying to stop time, ... quickly brings death into the present.'[13]

Anger

Another significant byproduct of anxiety is anger, which emerges out of spiritual disease and can become a basic driving force in a person's life. One author defined anger in this manner: 'Anger may best be described as a combination of uneasiness, discomfort, tenseness, resentment (which is response to selective stimuli), and frustration.'[14]

Most people would agree that they have experienced anger. There is likely less agreement about how anger is experienced, or how it is expressed. In his book on anger, L Madow notes that the expressions of anger fall into three categories. 'The first group is modified expressions of anger ... the second indirect expressions of anger, and the third variations of depression.'[15] In other words, anger can be expressed outwardly in either a controlled (modified) or uncontrolled (indirect) manner, or expressed inwardly in a way that wounds (depresses) the inner self. John Savage makes a similar observation when he speaks of anger as being either projected or repressed.

> The way in which people deal with anger varies considerably ... Anger may appear in the form of projection. In its extreme form it is seen as paranoia. If the anger is not conscious, the tendency is to act on that feeling rather than feeling it directly. This is commonly called 'acting out.'
>
> ... The other track is to turn the anger in on the self ... Displacement is the function of repressed anger, where, instead of acting out, the person 'acts in.' The result of 'acting in' is frequently seen as a conversion system in which ... psychosomatic disorders occur.[16]

Yet a third author notes that 'anger may be so threatening that it is either repressed (involuntary) or suppressed (voluntary).'[17]

In general those who study anger agree that it is dangerous. There are, of course, responses to anger that may be positive or benign. If controlled, and 'projected carefully,' anger may lead to beneficial action. A person, angry at a social injustice, may be moved to address that injustice. If 'suppressed,' and consciously not expressed (at least for the moment) it may be benign. It has been named and owned and it may be expressed in a controlled and non-destructive manner later. But all too frequently responses to anger are not beneficial. Anger is either repressed or it is allowed to express (or project) itself in an uncontrolled manner. Either way it is a force that brings harm to both the self and others. Projected, it wounds bodies, egos, emotions, and souls. Repressed, it eats away at the fabric of a person's being. Beuchner relates the insidious nature of anger in this way:

> Of the seven deadly sins anger is possibly the most fun. To lick your wounds, to smack your lips over grievances long past, to roll over your tongue the prospect of bitter confrontations still to come, to savor the last toothsome morsel both the pain you are given and the pain you are giving back – in many ways it is a feast fit for a king. The chief drawback is that what you are wolfing down is yourself. The skeleton at the feast is you.[18]

For many people anger is a significant barrier to wholeness. It is easy to understand how anger can damage the inner, the social, and the spiritual self, but the impact of anger on the physical self cannot be ignored. Returning to the concept of the inherent connectedness of all aspects of the person, what happens in one part of the self has an impact on all the other parts. A bodily wound has real impact on the social, soulful, spiritual self. In the same way, the ravages of anger, primarily present in the social realm or festering in the inner self, may well affect physical health, or hinder a person's capacity for healing.

Mr P was a 67-year-old man who spent the last 23 years of his life in a series of nursing homes. He had served with Patton's third army at the Battle of the Bulge in World War Two and returned home to work at a construction job in good health. In 1952, he suffered an injury on the job when he fell 60 feet from a bridge he was helping to build. He sustained a severe spinal cord injury, losing all use of his legs and most of the function in his arms. Since he had no family and was unable to care for himself, he was placed in a nursing home at the age of 44. Mr P was never able to get over the fact that he had survived the war only to suffer debilitating injury in an accident. He was angry at the construction company and the city and he was angry at God. Although never a religious man, he was convinced that God had not heard his prayers and that faith offered only a false hope. He was mean to the nurses who cared for him and disdainful of his many physicians. While moving in and out of nine different care facilities, he discovered how to smuggle whiskey into his room and began to drink heavily whenever he could. The nursing home staff was dismayed by his lack of respect for their rules and the staff often treated him poorly.

Six months before his death, Mr P was diagnosed with colon cancer. A series of meetings with his new physician resulted in a reduction in his hostility. He was given the opportunity to teach medical students about the challenge of caring for the disabled and was able to share his anger with the nursing home staff. He died in hospice care at his last nursing home. The staff held a memorial service for him after his death. No one attended but his care providers.

Guilt

When it comes to spiritual dis-ease, there is probably no issue more powerful than that of guilt. People often joke about guilt and its relationship to spirituality, or more frequently, religion. One man in Oregon jokingly calls himself a 'Zen Catholic.' Referring to his Irish Catholic background, which for him was the basis of some guilty feelings, he says, 'I not only feel guilt, I meditate on it.' Even the quirky comic strip Non Sequitur picks up this theme (*see* Figure 4.1).

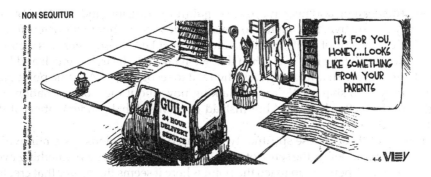

Figure 4.1

Non Sequitur © 1998 Wiley Miller. Distributed by Universal Press Syndicate, Inc. Reprinted with permission. All rights reserved.

It is an odd relationship. Spirituality is supposed to enhance life. It is supposed to give people strength, hope, understanding or wisdom, comfort, and meaning. Yet many of those who pursue spirituality, especially through the medium of organized religion, find that their spiritual life does not augment life but depletes it. They are left feeling inadequate, guilty, and in some cases even cursed. In one woman's words, 'I am not a good woman, although God knows I have tried. But trying has meant failing, it has meant falling short of God's plan. Now my life is chaos, I am abandoned by those I love. God has justly cursed my path and left me in darkness.'

Many authors have tried to address the issue of religion and guilt, and the provocative nature of the issue is even reflected in their titles: *Guilt, Where Theology and Psychology Meet;*[19] *'Guilt: Christian motivation or neurotic masochism?'*[20] One problem with guilt is that it is complex and diverse. It can be anything from a small twinge of regret to a powerful emotion that dominates life. It can drive people into immobility, or move them to change. It can be a positive factor, or negative.

One expert on guilt suggests that there are three types of guilt related integrally to three types of selves, which he identifies as the ideal self, the corrective self, and the punitive self.[21] The *ideal self* functions as the nucleus of conscience, and contains a person's values, standards, and aspirations. It might be said that the ideal self is an archetype as it serves as a measuring stick or ideal against which one measures behavior and, eventually, self-image. The activities of the *corrective self* are based upon the ideal self. The corrective self takes the person, with all of its thoughts, actions, and attitudes, and measures the real against the ideal. With the corrective self the ideal is appropriate, and the response to the 'corrections' are thoughtful and balanced. When a fault is found, the corrective self generates 'healthy guilt.' The internal voice or 'caregiver' reprimands the person who utilizes these reprimands in a self-reflective way. The inner corrective voice is the catalyst for examination, analysis, and change. The *punitive self* also measures the real against the ideal, but instead of providing appropriate corrections offers threats of punishment, rejection, or shaming. At this point a sense of 'wrongness' pervades one's being. A person has a sense of being flawed, essentially at odds with his or her true self.

This punitive self has also been called the 'critic.'[22] The critic is the negative and blaming voice inside a person's head that says, 'You're no good,' 'You're stupid,' 'What you're feeling is wrong,' or 'What you're trying to do will probably fail.' It can be so demeaning and negative that it is painful, confusing, and frightening. It is ultimately destructive, leading not to constructive change, but to more tension.

It is in this last type of guilt that the greatest danger lies. 'The danger of our guilt is less that we won't take it to heart than that we'll take it to heart too much and let it fester there in ways that we ourselves often fail to recognize.'[23] At some point guilt has morphed into shame. We are not talking now about the 'condemnation of a single, specific act or behavior' but instead of 'more global condemnation of the entire self.'[24]

For many of those whose spirituality is focused on a religious system in which there is a supreme being, the sense of guilt or shame can surface as something even darker, a curse. A person can reach the point where it seems the power that created and sustains the universe is terribly and irrevocably against them. They have sinned, failed, been wrong – indeed are wrong! And this wrongness has brought them inexorably to a place where nothing good can happen. This is not a neutral condition that has occurred through chance or fate. They are in a position of judgment because of their actions or their very nature. The extremity in which they now exit is a matter of accountability. They are cursed.

Ben was man in his mid-thirties. Ben's parents were conservative Christians and tended to believe that the best way to shape a young person was to point out anything that needed correcting. So they corrected, often. Unfortunately neither parent was particularly good at offering affection or affirmation. Ben grew up with a very healthy idea of what a 'good' person should be like, and a very firm conviction that he did not match this description. Indeed he reached a point where it seemed as if his best simply was not good enough – for his parents, and ultimately for God. Soon this negative spiritual thinking began to take control. Although Ben was a gifted person, and had been very successful by most standards, he still saw himself as flawed. Undeserving of praise, or success, he would frequently quote CS Lewis, noting that he was the lowest of the low, a tarnished object of scorn trapped in the 'ooze and slime and old decay.' He saw himself as cursed It was not just that he had slipped and thus found himself in the slime. God had pushed him into the muck, and was holding him down! His way of coping with this perception was twofold. Sometimes he simply failed to function. It was better to hold back and do nothing than to fail (although in fact he rarely failed at anything). In college, although an excellent athlete, he would fake injury to avoid 'making a fool' of himself. In other instances, when he had acted and succeeded, he would sabotage himself. He would do an excellent job at work, earn praise and promotion, and then secretly do something he considered evil. Finally, tired of fighting the battle between what he thought he was and what he should be, between the successful person he seemed to be on the outside and the failure he felt himself to be on the inside, he began to drink heavily. Eventually his worst dreams came true and he was fired from his job and humiliated in the eyes of his family and friends. He accepted his destruction, almost embraced it as his 'due.' Avoidance of his inner pain was not Ben's only negative coping mechanism. He not only tried to escape from his feelings into an alternate reality through substances, but he also attempted to simply avoid his feelings.

He shut down emotionally. Talking to Ben was like talking to a mask. He had little affect, showing a very small range of emotions outwardly. Many people praised him, saying he was 'amazingly calm,' but this calmness reflected an unwillingness to address the chaos within.

Ben's case demonstrates excessive or inappropriate guilt due to the assumption of unrealistic demands, initially created by his parents, but eventually self-generated. In other cases it is not so much that the demands are inappropriate, but that the person reacts in exaggerated ways to real or fancied transgression rather than simply accepting appropriate levels of responsibility. Having embraced his guilty feelings, Ben needed to deal with those feelings in some manner. Perhaps he needed to change his expectations. Or, if the situation was one where the expectation was appropriate, he needed to make amends to whoever had been violated, the sacred/divine, or another person. In Ben's case, these tasks remained incomplete. He did not revise his expectations, nor did he cope with his guilt appropriately. As a result, he reacted in a self-defeating manner and engaged in a form of self-punishment. This is not an unusual response to guilt.[25] In Ben's case this punishment was both conscious and unconscious. Punishment for guilt can be expressed in a variety of ways, somatically, emotionally, behaviorally, or even in the language of dreams.[26] Ben's response was heavily behavioral, although there was certainly an emotional component. In common language, he 'beat himself up.'

While guilt in moderate forms can serve some positive functions,[27] it is clear that when guilt is present at more extreme levels it can contribute to dis-ease and even mental illness. Guilt has been linked to Major Depressive Disorder and to Post-traumatic Stress Disorder.[28] While most authors who explore the impact of guilt feel it is pathological only in exaggerated or excessive forms, Albert Ellis goes so far as to insist that guilt is consistently pathological in nature.[29] A counter view to this is that of Tangey, who asserts that guilt is essentially non-pathological.[30] In the clinical setting it is most helpful to adopt the most common view, that guilt can be appropriate or inappropriate, moderate or extreme, helpful or destructive. In whatever form it emerges, guilt is a significant factor that affects people emotionally, socially, and spiritually.

Other issues

The list of spiritual 'issues' is long and varied. In addition to those already discussed, several others deserve mention, including fear, meaninglessness, and social disconnection. When people are in a state of spiritual dis-ease they fear many things. Fear can be extremely powerful, and have a negative impact up one's health, and one's ability to heal. Howard Clinebell suggests that fear is a major factor in the lives of people who are addictive, hooked on drugs, alcohol, work, or activity. 'If I keep myself half dead by guilt, compulsive work, unawareness, and worry, death is less threatening.'[31]

Another issue is meaninglessness, that 'Dark Night of the Soul' when one feels that all the things of this world have lost their appeal. One author describes the impact of meaninglessness, which is clearly an intense form of existential anxiety (Why do I exist?) in the following manner:

> Many addictions are attempts to escape from existential anxiety by centering life around a false absolute, by making a god of alcohol, food, work, drugs, or success. In this sense, addictions are forms of psychological idolatry. They are attempts to meet spiritual needs by non-spiritual means.[32]

When a person is in a state of spiritual disease, he/she becomes separated or disconnected from others, family, objects of love, even the sacred itself. Those who feel disconnected or abandoned often reflect that state in their relationships. A patient who has decided God doesn't care will often isolate him/herself. In the hospital they will simply turn away from others, facing the wall or a window. Those who feel abandoned by others, or who feel unworthy of affection, will actually disconnect emotionally from loved ones. They will stop talking, stop showing physical affection, refusing to hug or kiss. The family and friends of these people do not escape this general trend. In many cases a person who is in a state of spiritual dis-ease will project their sense of abandonment on their caregivers. They will become distrustful of their physicians, or nurses, or even the family member responsible for their ongoing care. They will be querulous and difficult to manage.

The impact of negative spiritual states

It is not unusual for healthcare professionals to struggle with the spiritual aspects of anxiety. Do hopelessness, helplessness, anger, and guilt cause anxiety or does unresolved anxiety cause these reactions? When is someone spiritually lost and when are they depressed? Does hopelessness cause depression or is it a symptom of depression? These questions reflect a linear model of thinking that forms the basis of traditional Western medicine, a model focused on the holy grail of cause and effect. But spiritual distress should not be thought of as a cause of mental illness. It is, instead, a different lens through which such patients can be understood. The physician can treat depression and still address spiritual wellness. Understanding spirituality adds to the physician's toolbox rather than replacing proven medical concepts. The spiritual dimension of health is not just another body system to assess for causation. It is an additional paradigm through which patients can be helped.

In an article authored in 1988 Albert Ellis provides an excellent illustration of the way spiritual issues may impact the attitudes and actions of the individual. He offers a list of eleven outcomes or characteristics. In this list Ellis repeatedly uses the word religion, but it is helpful to replace that word with the idea of 'spiritual distress' or 'spiritual dis-ease.' The list is as follows.[33]

1 Religion discourages self-acceptance.
2 Religion discourages self-interest.
3 Religion discourages self-directedness.
4 Religion tends to make healthy human-to-human relationships difficult.
5 Religion encourages intolerance of others.
6 Religion encourages inflexibility.
7 Religious people have difficulty accepting and living in the real world.
8 Religious people have difficulty accepting ambiguity and uncertainty.

9 Religious people use scientific thinking only until it conflicts with their religious beliefs, after which they begin thinking irrationally.

10 Religious people are prone to fanatical commitments, in contrast to emotionally health nonbelievers who commit passionately but not fanatically.

11 Emotionally stable people tend to be risk-takers in that they recognize what they want and take appropriate risks to achieve their goals; in contrast, religious people are too suffused with guilt to pursue their goals, because their world view requires self-sacrifice.

Ellis' list reflects many of the issues that have been discussed and can be related back to the three spiritual models as well as hopelessness, helplessness, anger, guilt, meaninglessness, and isolation or abandonment. It shows us that the negative impact of spiritual dis-ease can be expressed many ways, but reflects the consistency with which these major themes are addressed.

The part of a person that is spiritual can be incredibly significant in terms of wellness and should be addressed as a part of the therapeutic process. Lou Marinoff, reflecting upon what happens when people struggle philosophically with the big questions of life, refers to the negative impact of neglected spiritual stress.

> A dis-ease, if not eased, can eventually become a disease. It's much easier to treat a dis-ease with good ideas, before it escalates into disease and requires medical attention. A persistent state of dis-ease can taint or mar one's thoughts, words, and deeds – and will negatively affect one's emotional and physical well-being too.[34]

Spirituality as resource

A hospital chaplain, understanding the presence of spiritual issues and the powerful impact they have on people, developed a screening tool to help him assess spiritual health. What is impressive about his tool is the fact that it addresses both ends of the spiritual equation, the positive and the negative. This tool is based on the assumption that for every negative spiritual state there is an equally positive spiritual state. The concept assumes that peoples' spiritual lives are not static but dynamic, and that men and women move back and forth along a spectrum, between two opposite poles, depending upon circumstance and other factors.[35] A person can move from dis-ease to ease, from a spiritual emergency to spiritual stability. This model can be used easily by anyone who wants to explore the concept of spiritual issues, and reflect upon spiritual status. It is helpful for people to use their own terminology, terms that are meaningful to them, rather than just adopt the terms used by another. The very act of identifying spiritual issues and thinking about both positive and negative consequences is a process that can lead to spiritual awareness and growth. One possible set of themes follows.[36]

This model is a reminder that while, at times, spirituality is a therapeutic liability, it may also be a therapeutic asset. Many people benefit from the presence of their spiritual self and have a spirituality that is healthy. They are not spiritually distressed, or in a state of spiritual dis-ease, but are at peace. They are not disconnected, but profoundly connected to a source of power and hope. They are not stuck or lost, but have a sense of meaning and purpose in life that is not destroyed or shaken by tragedy or illness. And their spiritual thinking is healthy. They can put illness in the context of their spirituality in a manner that is appropriate and beneficial.

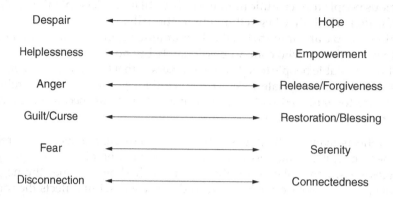

Figure 4.2

This model also illustrates that no spiritual state is permanent and that a person can move back and forth between spiritual distress and spiritual stability. A person who, because of negative spiritual thinking, sees herself as guilty and cursed, does not have to stay in that debilitating place, but can move across the spectrum to the point she believes that failure is not final and something good can and should happen in her life. A person who is trapped by fear in a position of dread can experience spiritual transformation, and become mobilized – still fearful, but able to cope with that fear and actively participate in life.

Because spirituality can be beneficial as well as harmful it is useful to move beyond the issues created by spiritual distress and explore the positive end of the spectrum. What are the themes when a person's spirituality is healthy? How does that healthy form of spirituality aid the therapeutic process?

Despair–hope

On the other end of the spectrum of hopelessness, what some might call despair, is hope. Hope involves a sense of future, a belief that there is something ahead. Being at peace spiritually, feeling connected to the sacred, believing one is 'on the way,' moving forward with purpose and direction, makes hope a viable option. In other words, one has belief that there is some reality that keeps him from the state of despair, or her from being overwhelmed by anxiety. This reality can be a god who acts in human history, the sacred, a philosophical system, nature, or science. It can even be a person, such as a counselor or mentor. It is often a combination of several of these 'realities.' Hope moves the person from a mindset that negates possibilities to one that creates or envisions possibilities.

A powerful illustration of the power of hope is the placebo effect, a phenomenon well documented by Shapiro and Benson. Those who support the placebo effect note that if one believes in something, in its potential to help, then that intervention will often have the desired effect. In drug tests, people who believe they are receiving a new drug, but actually receive a pill with no active ingredient, often still improve – sometimes at a rate comparable with the drug itself. Faith in God, nature, science, or the physician can have a similar effect.

Yahne and Miller, in the book *Integrating Spirituality into Practice*, break hope down into two basic components;[37] hope as will and hope as way. The concept of 'hope as will' focuses on the inner drive or desire to overcome. This can involve such victories as survival from an illness, victory over an obstacle, or advancement to a higher level of understanding. It involves the determination to keep learning, living, struggling, even in the face of tremendous barriers. It is the maintenance of dignity, and self-esteem even in the presence of disease or death. 'Hope as way' is less about an inner drive, and more about a hope-filled attachment to something or someone outside the self. With 'hope as way' people have hope *in* someone or something. This is the hope seen in the 12-step program of Alcoholics Anonymous, in the belief in a power outside of and greater than oneself that enables one to overcome addiction. This kind of hope accepts the limits of self-hope, perhaps even human hope in general, and focuses on a higher source of hope.

In some cases hope is very generalized. It is a relatively vague sense that 'things will get better', that there will be relief. In other instances, hope is much more specific. 'I hope I will recover from my illness.' 'I hope I can stop drinking.' 'I hope my marriage will survive.' Ideally hope is related to action. It is translated into following a treatment plan, even though the chances of success are very slim. It is expressed as a willingness to keep on loving and helping, even when one's own life is disintegrating. Hope, as an old saying goes, is the 'ants in the pants of faith.' It is so important that inspiring hope has been described as the practitioner's first duty to the client and a major contribution to treatment.[38]

> May is a 94-year-old woman who has enjoyed good health her entire life. Along with her supportive family, she visited her family physician to complain about fatigue and loss of energy. A medical evaluation discovered a severe anemia caused by ongoing blood loss in her stool and a subsequent endoscopic test found a large colon cancer. May's family was concerned that she might not survive surgical removal of the tumor at her age. But after extended discussion, May elected to proceed with an operation. She told her physicians that she had enjoyed a wonderful life and was at peace regardless of the outcome. But she knew in her heart that things would turn out 'as they were meant to be.' Her surgery went well and she recovered her usual level of function within six weeks of the operation. May knows that her tumor may return, but she has an abiding hope that her life's work is not yet complete.

Helplessness–empowerment

For some, there is a powerful sense that there is nothing they can do. The illness, the addiction, the situation is simply beyond current resources; the problem is without a possible solution. This person may have still have a sense of hope, which transcends the situation, but the immediate scenario itself is beyond redemption. For example, a person may have a sense that his situation is helpless, he is going to die of his disease, but a corresponding sense of hopefulness, that there will be a life after death, or that even in the face of death, love can be found. The issue here is empowerment. The opposite of helplessness is thus empowerment, the sense that one can, in fact, facilitate change. Spirituality can clearly impact a person's sense of empowerment. It can develop one's inner power, and/or it can connect a person to an external power, to someone or something greater than one's self.

From a therapeutic perspective, helplessness is a big problem. People who feel helpless are not likely to be active participants in the healing process. Such patients may be non-compliant, and overly passive. After all, what difference does it make, they are helpless to initiate change. The empowered person, no matter how difficult the situation, still believes that something can be done. There are always possibilities. A person can know that they are going to die, and that they are powerless to change that reality, but they may still believe in their personal power to create something positive within that difficult context. They may work with their healing team to extend life, or may seek to make the life that remains as productive and rich as possible. They will ignore what they cannot do and seek to find activities they can do.

Shirley, who was in her mid-sixties, was, after years of vague and confusing symptoms, diagnosed with bulbar palsy. The prognosis was without hope. This debilitating disease would continue to attack her nervous system, rendering her ever more disabled. At first Shirley was overwhelmed with helplessness. She was inclined to believe there was nothing she could do to make life better, no way she could contribute. What made the situation worse was the fact that Shirley was a doer, not a talker. She had always had difficulty expressing her feelings to other people, and preferred to show her love by doing things for others. She had been extremely active in her community, and was known for everything from community leadership to holiday dessert boxes. Fortunately her family physician understood the issue. He encouraged her to think of things she would like to do that she had not done. 'I'd like to travel,' Shirley responded, 'but I can't.' In the end Shirley decided to take each of her three children on a trip. It would be a gift to herself, allowing her to complete trips that she and her now-deceased husband had planned to take together. But it was also something she could do for her children. She was not powerless.

It is hard to estimate the impact the transformation from helpless to empowerment had on Shirley's illness, but most of those around her believed that it not only gave her additional energy, and additional days, perhaps years, but that it gave her a much higher quality of life as well.

Anger–forgiveness

Anger, which has been seen to be an incredibly destructive emotion, is balanced by the concepts of forgiveness and/or reconciliation. Forgiveness is a spiritual discipline. One author defines forgiveness as 'a willingness to abandon one's right to resentment, negative judgment, and an indifferent behavior toward someone who unjustly injured us.'[39] Another author notes that forgiveness relates 'specifically to a change in emotion,'[40] observing that the root of the word means to give up or give away anger and its accompanying actions, revenge, and retribution. The word's origins, the authors insist:

> ...reflect its centrality to human relations and human's life in community. Without the ability to let go of anger, life would be hell. Take a moment to imagine the state of one's life if one could neither forgive

nor expect forgiveness for the hurts, wrongs, or disappointments given and received. One would be caught in perpetual punishment, personal despair, social chaos and war.[41]

Forgiveness is an act of will, which often involves a difficult process that extends over time. It is not forgetting an event, or its impact on the self, but processing that event, feeling the pain, and then letting go of it. 'To forgive an act does not mean to pretend it never existed. Instead forgiveness involves preventing the act from controlling one's every waking moment.'[42] It is a critical step to moving on with life. Kabat-Zinn's mediation guide *Wherever You Go, There You Are*[43] illustrates well the fact that the baggage people carry with them, including unresolved anger, affects life in profound ways. Unresolved anger drags people down, keeping them from connecting with others, and from moving forward on the quest for life and meaning. Forgiveness, letting go of the anger, frees one to connect with others in meaningful ways. It may even lead to reconciliation, to a rebuilding of the relationship with the person who caused the anger in the beginning. Forgiveness also allows a person to move on, unencumbered, into the future.

Charlie is a 56-year-old man who has experienced depression and poor sleep for four years. His symptoms began after his small business was robbed and he was beaten by the young man who committed the robbery. Charlie's physical injuries were minor, but he felt violated and experienced profound anger about the attack. He took self-defense courses and purchased a handgun to protect himself from future attacks. His personal and business relationships suffered as bitterness permeated his relationships. Finally, after being confronted by his wife, Charlie visited his attacker in prison and learned about the young man's struggle with drug addiction. He decided to volunteer at a drug treatment program and began to sleep better. His relationships improved. Charlie finally became able to understand his attack as a turning point in his life and that the changes in him were positive.

Research indicates that the practice of forgiveness is beneficial, and can be related to such benefits as a decrease in depression, anxiety, and hostility in both men and women.[44] Since forgiveness involves letting go of anger, it not only helps repair broken relationships, but enhances the overall capacity of people to develop and maintain healthy relationships.

Obviously there are times when the person who must be forgiven is one's self (*see* 'Guilt' above). In these times, one must not only let go of anger at one's self, but one must move toward reconciliation with the one harmed. Sanderson and Linehan suggest the following guidelines for reconciliation, based upon the research literature around this issue.[45]

1 Give a sincere and validating apology.
2 If possible, repair the hurt.
3 Commit to not engage in the injurious behavior again.
4 Follow through on the commitment by changing the behavior.
5 Engage in conciliatory acts.

Forgiveness is powerful. It can bring release, freedom, and reconciliation. It involves not only letting go of the past, but also investing in the future. It is a worthy foil to anger, one of the most powerful of the negative spiritual states.

> When somebody you've wronged forgives you, you're spared the dull and self-diminishing throb of a guilty conscience. When you forgive somebody who has wronged you, you're spared the dismal corrosion of bitterness and wounded pride. For both parties, forgiveness means the freedom again to be at peace inside their own skins and to be glad in each other's presence.[46]

Guilt–restoration

The other end of the spectrum of guilt would be restoration or blessing – arriving at the point where one still admits that he or she was wrong, but is able to process that failure, let go of it, and move on. It is not a process that happens quickly or easily. In thinking about the spectrum of guilt and acceptance it is helpful to think in terms of what acceptance is not. It is not repression, stuffing the feelings of guilt down and ignoring their presence. It is not denial, convincing one's self that what occurred was not really wrong or didn't really happen. It is not deflection, finding someone else to be the focus of blame for what occurred.

Acceptance first involves the act of ownership. One must 'own' the error and admit the guilt. Consider the prodigal son in the Christian Bible. This man had clearly erred, having taken his inheritance and 'squandered his wealth in wild living' (Luke 15:13). Eventually, however, after sinking so low that he ended up feeding pigs, an animal considered unclean by his faith system, he came to a point when he 'owned' his misbehavior and saw himself for who he really was. This step of owning his error was the beginning of a process of reconciliation and healing. Humble and contrite, he returned to his father, whose generosity he had violated, and said, 'Father, I have sinned against heaven and against you. I am no longer worthy to be called your son' (Luke 15:21). The father, sensing the authenticity of the son's contrition, forgave him and restored him to the family.

Second, there is the need to sort out and perhaps repair the situation. Part of this process may involve exploring how the behavior is in conflict with personal values. 'Value-behavior incongruencies may be one of the defining characteristics of humankind in that all human beings experience conflict between their behavior and their expressed values from time to time in their lives.'[47] A person must ask, 'How did I violate my values? How did that violation impact me, or others? How do I feel about that violation?' The real issue is whether the person, after asking the tough questions, and confronting the tough answers, can resolve the situation and keep it from contributing to emotional problems.

Third, there is acceptance, a need to embrace the guilt. This means simply to acknowledge the impact of the error and the feelings, hurt, and anger attached to the guilt-producing behavior. Acceptance is not for the weak or fainthearted. It can be painful and disturbing. But by facing the behavior, the healing process begins.

Eventually this process leads to healing, reconciliation, and change (restoration). Guilt can motivate a person to examine life, to explore beliefs and values. It can be the beginning of change. This is a key part of the healing process as defined by the 12-step program. Several steps require acknowledgment of error, and disclosure of those misbehaviors (steps 4, 5, and 10). But the person is asked to do more than just recognize and share the guilt, they are asked to make amends (steps 8–10). They must work to right the wrongs. They must tell those they have hurt about their 'good grief' and attempt to do something corrective and constructive.

As has been recognized by Alcoholics Anonymous (AA), moving from guilt to acceptance can be very important to the therapeutic process. A person who has resolved guilt has released emotional baggage. They have learned to develop relationships based on honesty, respect, and the ability to admit and resolve wrongdoings. They have become stronger and more congruent. All of these things are benefits to the person who is struggling with either disease or dis-ease.

Fear or discontent–serenity

In many cases people who are ill are inwardly chaotic and gripped by fear. Those who are struggling with guilt are not at peace with their past. Those struggling with fear, or discontent, are not at peace with their present or their future. On the opposite end of the spectrum from fear is a state where spiritual thinking is positive and people tend to experience what we call serenity. This state is effectively expressed in The Serenity Prayer.

> God, grant me the serenity to accept the things I cannot change,
> The courage to change the things I can,
> And the wisdom to know the difference.
>
> Living one day at a time,
> Enjoying one moment at a time,
> Accepting hardship as a pathway to peace
> Taking this sinful world as it is,
> Not as I would have it.
>
> Trusting that you will make all things right
> If I surrender to your will,
> So that I may be reasonably happy in this life
> And supremely happy with you forever in the next.

This prayer, often attributed to Reinhold Niebuhr, but most likely the work of a little-known eighteenth-century theologian, suggests that serenity is courage, peace, patience, acceptance, and trust. It is being in touch with reality, no matter how painful, but still essentially at peace, functional, even joyful, no matter what that reality might be.

Several years ago, researchers exploring the concept of serenity in gerontology came up with 10 characteristics that they believe define serenity. Those characteristics are:

1 The ability to detach from desires and/or emotion and feelings.
2 The ability to be in touch with an inner haven of peace and security.
3 A sense of connectedness with the universe.
4 A trust in the wisdom of the universe.
5 The habit of actively pursuing all reasonable avenues for solving problems.
6 An ability to accept situations that cannot be changed.
7 A way to give unconditionally of one's self.

8 Forgiveness of self and others.

9 The ability to let go of the past and the future and to live in the present.

10 A sense of perspective as to the importance of one's self and life events.[48]

It is easy to see how these characteristics would contribute to the therapeutic process. A person who is serene is free from the past and will not be burdened by guilt and shame. They are confident about the future, believing in themselves, other people, the nature of the universe, and in the divine or sacred. And they are comfortable with the present, able to cope effectively with what is occurring in their lives.

Agnes was a woman in her seventies who had been diagnosed with pancreatic cancer. By the time the tumor was discovered the illness was relatively advanced and she was given little time to live. Agnes spent a great deal of time in pain. Although her physician attempted to control the pain, Agnes was reluctant to take much medication, and thus was often uncomfortable. However Agnes had a well-developed ability to cope. In her worst moments, she would retreat inside. She had a special phrase, she hesitated to call it a mantra, that she would chant. She would concentrate on the words, on the rhythm, and ultimately on God, and, as she described it, 'move beyond the pain.' Her phrase was the Jewish saying – baruch attar adonai, 'blessed be the Lord.' Agnes knew she was going to die. She had no illusions about the reality and seriousness of her illness, but in a remarkable way she refused to allow the cancer to define her. She continued to sing in the choir. A musician, she donated her Steinway grand piano to the church, and insisted that she be the first to play it in its new setting. She started a calling campaign, calling others in her local congregation afflicted by cancer to give them words of encouragement. Her answer to those who wondered why she was supporting people who were, in many cases, less ill than she, was curt: 'because I've got something to give.' Agnes died only a few months after her diagnosis. But she left an indelible mark on the community that surrounded her.

What we see in Agnes is a number of benefits emerging from a healthy spirituality. We see an ability to find an inner haven. Instead of being dominated by what was occurring in her life, what has happened in the past, and what might happen in the future, Agnes turned to a 'safe place.' In her case that place was in the presence of a loving God. We also see an ability to accept not only the current reality, which is beyond control, but also the self. Agnes was comfortable enough with who she was to enjoy her unique abilities and inherent value. Out of this self-acceptance came an ability to embrace others.

Sylvia Boorstein, while reflecting upon a time when she was confronted with the unchangeable, the news that her father had untreatable cancer, explored the concept of chaos versus peace. She illustrates powerfully the difference between spiritual health and spiritual disease. Spiritual health is marked by a mind free of chaos, tension, constrictions. Spiritual illness is marked by a mind crowded and tangled with fears and tensions.

> The mind free of tension is spacious. Actually the mind is always spacious – its essence is seamless spaciousness – tangles of tensions ... cause it to feel restricted. The tensions cause suffering. The tensions are suffering. For me, the word 'soft' also works well. The mind free of tensions is soft. Malleable. It absorbs shocks.[49]

The person who has moved from chaos and fear to peace is the one whose spiritual life has created a spacious, soft, and supple mind.

Another possible version of this particular spectrum involves the use of the words 'curse' and 'blessing.' For the person who is in the realm of curse, life is all fear. This person sees little opportunity for good, little chance of a good outcome. Dark events are final and define life. For the person who is in the realm of blessing there is always a sense that good is present. Even in the darkness of illness, injury, disability, and impending death, life can be a blessing, a gift.

Disconnected–connected

It is remarkable how many spiritual issues involve some sort of relationship. It is very clear how debilitating it is to feel disconnected, from one's self, from others, and from the sacred. 'To be lonely is to be aware of an emptiness which it takes more than people to fill. It is to sense that something is missing that you cannot name.'[50]

It is also clear how empowering and calming it is to be connected and to know that there is someone or something there. The benefits of connection – feeling loved and valued, listened to and encouraged, accepted as one is, forgiven, having a sense that help is available – all aid the therapeutic process.

A person who feels connected trusts, and is far more likely to trust and value, those, such as nurses and physicians, who are part of the healing process. A connected person has hope, and remains responsive, open to possibilities and blessings. A connected person believes there is help, and does not become frozen and immobilized by powerlessness. A connected person can let go of the past, drop the baggage of guilt, and move forward more freely, ready to repent, to change, to live life in a new way. The connected personality can have serenity and live in the moment and for the moment, making the most of each day, each hour, each minute.

The power of connection is powerfully voiced by Henri Nouwen when he suggests that being in the presence of hospitality, a welcoming presence:

> means primarily the creation of a free space where the stranger can enter and become a friend instead of an enemy. Hospitality is not to change people, but to offer them space where change can take place... The paradox of hospitality is that it wants to create emptiness, not a fearful emptiness, but a friendly emptiness where the stranger can enter and discover themselves as created free; free to sing their own songs, speak their own languages, dance their own dances...[51]

When people are in the presence of the sacred, when they are in that free and friendly space, they can cope. More than that, they can discover, and grow, and celebrate, even in the wasteland of illness.

Thoughts for reflection

- As you think about the negative impact of an unhealthy spirituality, which issue or theme do you struggle with the most?
- When it comes to the positive impact of a healthy spirituality, which of the themes do you believe reflects your greatest spiritual strength?

Notes

1 Fisher D. *From Maintenance to Recovery: how consumers are transforming the mental health system*. A talk given to the Association of Oregon Community Mental Health Programs, September 29, 2004, Hood River, Oregon. Quote used with permission.

2 'Disease' relates to a physical, biomedical condition. 'Dis-ease' refers to inner turmoil emerging from or focused in the emotion, spiritual, or relational. The term 'illness' encompasses the entire complex, disease and dis-ease alike.

3 Savage J (1976) *The Bored and Apathetic Church Member*. LEAD Consultants, Pitford, NY, p.3.

4 Engles GL (1962) *Psychological Development in Health and Disease*. WB Saunders Co., Philadelphia, PA, p.168.

5 Engles GL (1962) *Psychological Development in Health and Disease*. WB Saunders Co., Philadelphia, PA, p.168.

6 Tillich P (1956) *The Courage to Be*. Yale University Press, New Haven, CT, p.35.

7 Tillich P (1957) *Systematic Theology, Vol II*. University of Chicago Press, Chicago, IL, pp.534, 535–6.

8 Heidegger M (1963) *Being and Time*. Harper & Row, New York, NY, pp.1–438.

9 Kierkegaard S (trans. Walter Lowrie) (1944) *The Concept of Dread*. Princeton Press, Princeton, NJ.

10 Savage J (1976) *The Bored and Apathetic Church Member*. LEAD Consultants, Pitford, NY, p.6.

11 Savage J (1976) *The Bored and Apathetic Church Member*. LEAD Consultants, Pitford, NY, p.6.

12 Claypool J (1974) *Tracks of a Fellow Struggler*. Word, Waco, TX, p.95.

13 Rush AK (1973) *Getting Clear: body work for women*. Random House, New York, NY, p.281.

14 Stern FR (1972) *Anger, Psychology, Physiology, Pathology*. Charles C. Thomas, Springfield, IL, p.5.

15 Madow L (1972) *Anger*. Charles Scribner's Sons, New York, NY, pp.5–7.

16 Savage J (1976) *The Bored and Apathetic Church Member*. LEAD Consultants, Pitford, NY, pp.25–7.

17 Lidz T (1968) *The Person*. Basic Books, Inc., New York, NY, p.257.

18 Buechner F (1973) *Wishful Thinking*. Harper & Row, New York, NY, p.2.

19 Narramore SB (1974) Guilt: where theology and psychology meet. *Journal of Psychology and Theology*. **2**: 18–25.

20 Narramore SB (1974) Guilt: Christian motivation or neurotic masochism? *Journal of Psychology and Theology*. **2**: 182–9.

21 Narramore SB (1974) Guilt: where theology and psychology meet. *Journal of Psychology and Theology*. **2**: 18–25.

22 Gendlin ET (1961) Experiencing: a variable in the process of therapeutic change. *American Journal of Psychotherapy*. **15**: 233–45.

23 Beuchner F (1973) *Wishful Thinking*. Harper & Row, New York, NY, pp.34–5.

24 Faiver C, Ingersoll RE, O'Brien E and McNally C (2001) *Explorations in Counseling and Spirituality.* Thomson Learning – Brooks/Cole, Belmont, CA, p.76.

25 Osborne C (1967) *The Art of Understanding Yourself.* Zondervan, Grand Rapids, MI.

26 Drakeford JW (1967) *Integrity Therapy.* Broadman Press, Nashville, TN.

27 Ferguson TJ and Crowley SL (1997) Measure for measure: a multitrait-multimethod analysis of guilt and shame. *Journal of Personality Assessment.* **69**: 425–41.

28 Faiver C, Ingersoll RE, O'Brien E and McNally C (2001) *Explorations in Counseling and Spirituality.* Thomson Learning – Brooks/Cole, Belmont, CA, p.78.

29 Ellis A (1980) Psychotherapy and atheistic values: a response to A.E. Bergin's 'Psychotherapy and Religious Values'. *Journal of Consulting and Clinical Psychology.* **48**: 635–9.

30 Tangey JP (1990) Assessing individual differences in proneness to shame and guilt: development of the self-conscious affect and attribution inventory. *Journal of Anxiety Disorders.* **5**: 359–67.

31 Clinebell H (1979) *Growth Counseling.* Abingdon, Nashville, TN, p.110.

32 Stotland E (1969) *The Psychology of Hope.* Jossey-Bass, San Francisco, CA, p.21–2.

33 Ellis A (1988) Is religiosity pathological? *Free Inquiry.* **18**: 27–32.

34 Marinoff L (2003) *Therapy for the Sane.* Bloomsbury, New York, NY, p.12.

35 Hodges S (1999) Spiritual screening: the starting place for intentional pastoral care. *Chaplaincy Today.* **15**(1): 30–9.

36 This set of themes is that developed by Dr Stephen Kliewer, one of the co-authors of this book. The concept is based upon the work of S Hodges.

37 Miller WR (ed.) (1999) *Integrating Spirituality into Treatment.* American Psychological Association, Washington DC, pp.220–2.

38 Pipher M (1996) *The Shelter of Each Other: rebuilding our families.* Ballantine Books, New York, NY. As noted in Miller WR (ed.) (1999) *Integrating Spirituality into Treatment.* American Psychological Association, Washington DC, p.224.

39 Enright RD, Freedman S and Risque J (1988) The psychology of interpersonal forgiveness. In: RD Enright and J North (eds) *Exploring Forgiveness.* University of Wisconsin Press, Madison, WI, pp.46–9.

40 Miller WR (ed.) (1999) *Integrating Spirituality into Treatment.* American Psychological Association, Washington DC, p.207.

41 Miller WR (ed.) (1999) *Integrating Spirituality into Treatment.* American Psychological Association, Washington DC, pp.207, 208.

42 Faiver C, Ingersoll RE, O'Brien E and McNally C (2001) *Explorations in Counseling and Spirituality.* Thomson Learning – Brooks/Cole, Belmont, CA, p.32.

43 Kabat-Sinn J (1994) *Wherever You Go, There You Are.* Hyperion, New York, NY.

44 Coyle CT and Enright RD (1997) Forgiveness intervention with postabortion men. *Journal of Consulting and Clinical Psychology.* **65**: 1042–6.

45 Sanderson C and Linehan MM (1999) Acceptance and forgiveness. In: WR Miller (ed.) *Integrating Spirituality into Treatment.* American Psychological Association, Washington DC, pp.212–13.

46 Beuchner F (1973) *Wishful Thinking.* Harper & Row, New York, NY, p.29.

47 Miller WR (ed.) *Integrating Spirituality into Treatment.* American Psychological Association, Washington DC, p.151.

48 Roberts K and Cunningham G (1990) Serenity: concept analysis and measurement. *Educational Gerontology.* **16**: 577–89. Quoted in Miller WR (ed.) (1999) *Integrating Spirituality into Treatment.* American Psychological Association, Washington DC, p.239.

49 Boorstein S (1998) *That's Funny, You Don't Look Buddhist.* HarperCollins, New York, NY, pp.35–6.

50 Buechner F (1988) *Whistling in the Dark: a theological ABC.* Harper & Row, San Francisco, CA, pp.75–6.

51 Nouwen H (1975) *Reaching Out.* Doubleday, New York, NY, p.51.

CHAPTER 5

The culture of one

I know you think you understand what you heard me say. But I don't
think you understand that what you heard was not what I said.

Unknown

Communication is a basic life skill. Our ability to communicate significantly affects
our ability to be successful in life. It not only affects our ability to apply skills
effectively in a work environment, but it facilitates the capacity to build deep and
lasting relationships. Communication is the bridge over which not only information, but also emotion and concern move from person to person. Communication is how people connect. The more important the focus of the communication,
the more profoundly a person feels about the thoughts and feelings being expressed, the more critical it is that the communication process be effective. The
more important the focus of the communication, the more profound and complex
the issues being discussed, the more difficult communication seems to be. When
talking about truly critical issues, such as health, life, death, and spirituality, it is
difficult for people to say what they mean, to present a clear, direct message. When
one listens to people share their thoughts and feelings about such topics, it is
difficult to really hear.

The art of communication is a key component to the practice of medicine in
general and the integration of spirituality and healthcare in particular. First, these
skills will enable us to help people say what they mean, even when talking about
powerful and sometimes painful issues. It will help move them from indirect
expressions to direct expressions. Second, communication skills will help us draw
forth, often from the depths of the person, thoughts, feelings, and perceptions that
may be hindering the process of healing. Sometimes the patient is aware of these
feelings and issues and has chosen not to express them, generally as a protective
strategy. At other times they may be only vaguely aware of these internal dynamics,
and may, in some cases, be essentially unaware that these feelings and issues exist.
Third, communication becomes a therapeutic tool that facilitates problem solving,
the exploration of issues, and other critical tasks. Communication is not only a basic
life skill, but it is the basic tool for the integration of spirituality and healthcare.

The struggle to communicate

Much of the problem lies in the nature of communication itself. Communication
involves two basic steps. First there must be output, what is usually referred to as
'talking,' and second there must be input, what is normally called listening. This
seems simple enough at first glance, but in fact this process is extremely complex
and difficult. It is made difficult by what might be called the 'Interpersonal Gap.'

We can understand this gap if we look at a cognitive map of the interaction between two people. Any interaction takes two separate personages, both of whom are incredibly unique. Each of these people has their own thoughts, ideas, inferences, and experiences that make them who they are.

In order to communicate with the other, one of the people has to take what is inside, and can only be known directly by himself/herself, and make it public. The emotions, ideas, and thoughts that are within have to be 'encoded' so that others have access to them. This process of encoding usually involves three basic domains – words, body language, and tone of voice. The second person has to 'decode' this communication. The exchange can be illustrated as shown in Figure 5.1.

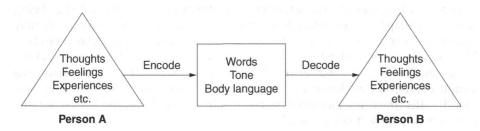

Figure 5.1

The first thing to note is that what is inside and private, known only to the person himself/herself, must be made public. It must be translated into a medium accessible to others. This means that whatever is expressed by our 'encoder' is in fact 'in code,' and thus to some degree indirect. The major three mediums through which communications are expressed are words, tone of voice, and body language. According to Dr Albert Mehrabian, a Professor of Communications who pioneered communications research in the 1960s, most of our communication is not, as is often assumed, expressed through our words. Instead it is often the other facets of our encoding systems that are the most powerful. Mehrabian suggested that when a person puts inner thoughts and feelings into a public medium, 7% of the meaning is in the words that are spoken, 38% of the meaning is paralinguistic, contained in the way that the words are said (tone of voice), and 55% of meaning is found in facial expression and body language.[1] Behavior or actions can also be added to the non-verbal (body language) mix.

The fact that the expressions of a person's inner thoughts, feelings, and intentions must be put into such codes can create significant problems. A major problem that can occur during the 'encoding' process is incongruence. Incongruence materializes when a person sends a message and the content of the three major domains (words, tone, and body language) aren't consistent. For example, if a person states that they are 'not angry,' but their tone of voice and body language clearly seem to indicate that they are, we have incongruence. Incongruence can occur for a number of reasons. It can be intentional, with a person consciously saying what they do not mean. Many people simply cannot present a congruent message if they are being deceitful. They will say one thing, but their tone of voice or body language will almost always betray them. Of course there are people who can state a falsehood and still make all the aspects of their communication match. But while congruence is no guarantee of honesty, it certainly provides an important clue. It should be noted that the general rule is to put the most trust in that facet of communication over which people have the least control. Using this rule, words, which are the most controllable, are to be trusted least, and body language, especially such clues as muscular tension, flushing, and sweating, are to be trusted the most.

Of course incongruence can also occur unintentionally, usually when a person does not really understand what is going on in the inner person. Perhaps they are angry, but have failed to recognize that anger. So they will say, quite honestly, that they are not angry, but their tone and body language will reveal the anger that is really there.

Incongruence can also occur because of factors outside a person's control. For example, a person's facial structure may mislead those who interact with him/her. A person with a mouth that naturally turns down may be interpreted as being 'dour' or 'unhappy' when in fact they feel just fine. A person who flushes easily may be seen as embarrassed or angry when he/she is not feeling any strong emotion at all. Not only can there be 'encoding' errors that create confusion and misinterpretation, there can also be 'decoding' errors. It must be remembered that the person has within themselves all kinds of thoughts, experience, and inferences that profoundly affect the way a message is received or interpreted. Figure 5.2 is a schematic of how an interaction takes place.[2]

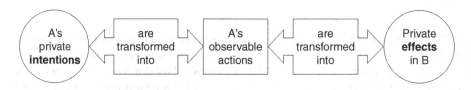

Figure 5.2

This process includes two transformations – the transformation from inner thoughts, reflections, intentions, and inferences into observable medium, and the transformation from the observable (seen and heard) medium back into an internal interpretation or effect. In effect both people in the process are imprinting their own unique personhood on the process during the transformation process. Because of this, both people are also 'guessing' or 'inferring' about what is actually happening during the transaction. 'B' is having to infer, based upon his/her interpretation of what is seen and heard, what 'A' intended to communicate. 'A', on the other hand, must infer, based upon how 'B' responds, whether the intended message was really received, and how that message affected the other person. Neither really knows directly what is going on within the other. And the more 'indirect' or vague the outward message is, the more tenuous the assumptions or inferences.

The uncertainty around this process is profound. Not only are people different, but so are their 'encoding' and 'decoding' processes. The result is that the same intentions may be expressed in significantly different actions, words, and tones; different intentions may be expressed by the same actions, words, and tones; the same words, actions, or tones may lead to different effects; different actions, words, and tones may lead to the same effects.

Martha was a young woman from a poor family who was married to a man from a rather affluent family. Because of her background experiences, which included never owning new clothes, living in a home furnished with battered furniture, and living in a relatively chaotic and unclean environment, she was extremely sensitive about her home and her housekeeping abilities. Her mother-in-law was a woman whose house was outstanding, not only for the quality of its ornamentation but for its organization and cleanliness. This intensified her feelings of insecurity and she was always extremely anxious when the 'in-laws' came to visit. The mother-in-law, for her part, was a person who had a great deal of difficulty expressing emotions. Her way of 'encoding' her feelings for people was to do nice things for them. Although she had rarely said 'I love you' to her children, she had worked hard to provide the best meals and the best clothes possible. She had served as a volunteer and had been very active in their lives. When visiting her daughter-in-law she wanted to communicate her affection so would turn to her natural method of expressing affection, doing something, specifically cleaning. Her focus was normally the kitchen, so she would move the refrigerator and clean behind it, clean the oven, and provide that 'extra' level of cleanliness so difficult to maintain in a busy household full of children. She would try to praise Martha, commenting on the 'interesting' (for her a very positive word) decorations. Martha, with her background and insecurities, did not receive the message that was intended. Instead, in the decoding process, she changed the message of affection to one of judgment. In the cleaning efforts of her mother-in-law she saw tacit disapproval of her cleaning efforts, and in the praise she heard condescension. Instead of feeling cared for she felt put down.

We can diagram the interchange between Martha and her mother-in-law (Andrea) as shown in Figure 5.3.

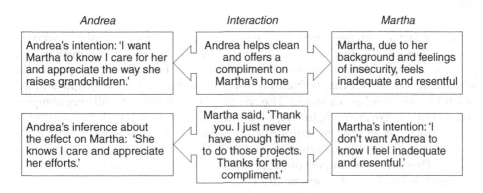

Figure 5.3

Note the difference between Andrea's intention and Martha's inference about Andrea's intention. Not only do they not match, they are almost opposites. The same disparity is present with respect to the effect of Andrea's 'message' on Martha and Andrea's inference about the effect on Martha.

This little interchange reflects well the complexity and challenge of the communication process. There are just too many variables – differences in how things are expressed, how the public message is delivered, and how the messages are interpreted. And there are critical differences in the people sending and receiving the message. It is, perhaps, this final difference that has the greatest impact on the process. Differences, in background, culture, or experience, function as lenses or prisms through which the messages must pass. Each time the message passes through a lens it is distorted, at least a little. It becomes, in most cases, less direct, less clear. If we think about the potential number of differences possible between two people, it is amazing that any message ever gets through. One good way to identify the lenses through which we send and receive messages is to think about all of the things that make us unique as a person. 'What is it about me that makes me unique, who I am?' During one rotation the Family Medicine residents at Oregon Health and Science University in Portland, Oregon, are asked to list the factors that make them unique. The words illustrating these factors are written on a board between two faces. As the residents explore this idea the board quickly becomes full, and a graphic illustration of why communication is difficult is created.

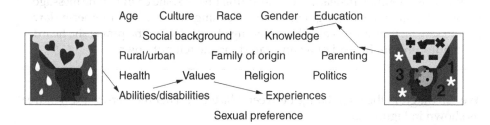

Figure 5.4

We are, in fact, all unique, with our own set of unique factors that make us who we are. Some of these factors are environmental, created by our life experiences, our parents, and other such influences. Other factors may be inherent, just part of the way we are 'wired.' We may be 'naturally' introverted or extroverted, right-brained or left-brained, thinkers or feelers. The critical point is that we are all very complex and all unique. We are each, in fact, a 'culture of one.' So not only is the communication process itself fraught with difficulties, but the process is made even more complicated by all those distinctive elements that make each of us unique and special. Those elements impact our ability to express messages clearly and hear the thoughts and feelings of others accurately.

As was noted earlier, the problems we have communicating with one another are made more intense when the subject of the interchange is something of great importance to either party. It is not nearly as difficult to talk about the weather as it is to talk about a moral or spiritual issue. It is harder to express our message clearly because topics such as spirituality touch the core of who we are, and revealing our thoughts and feelings about our spiritual life makes us vulnerable. It is harder to hear the message of another when such topics are discussed because the intensity of our own feelings about the issues affects our ability to receive the other's thoughts and feelings cleanly. We hear the other's words in the context of our own beliefs and cherished values. Sometimes this means we don't really hear them at all.

Implications for integration of spirituality and healthcare

This chapter began with the assertion that communication is a basic life skill. In the book *Messages*[3] the authors make some radical declarations about its importance.

> Your ability to communicate largely determines your personal happiness. When you communicate effectively you make and keep friends. You are valued at work. Your children respect and trust you. You get your sexual needs met... Effective communication makes life work.[4]

What has been learned both about the importance of communication and its complexity are instructive as one thinks about the integration of spirituality and healthcare. From the previous discussion the following principles emerge.

- First, each person is a culture of one. If we are to work with a person in a deep way, we must begin to understand their unique culture and avoid the trap of stereotypes.
- Second, if we are to be able to understand another's unique culture, and the forces that have shaped and continue to shape them, we must understand our own unique culture. It must be remembered that our personal culture powerfully affects the way we receive the messages of another.
- Third, if we would move with people into the realm of the spiritual, we must understand that each person also has a unique set of spiritual beliefs or values. They endow illness and healing with different meanings, depending on their unique spiritual culture. What does this person believe? How does he/she think about illness, health, healing, and the sacred? We cannot assume, because we know what faith system this person participates in, that we know their spiritual culture. We must respect the fact that there are infinite varieties of belief and an infinite number of ways to express belief. If we would enjoy the privilege of engaging with another at the level of spirituality we must explore their unique culture and learn to work within that framework.
- Fourth, if we would discover people's unique spiritual values, we must learn how to listen. This is the key to the effective integration of spirituality and healthcare.

Our personal cultures

A small-town doctor once found himself struggling to like one of his patients. There was no clear reason why he would dislike this person, but he found himself responding negatively to the patient, and being more critical and less compassionate than normal. Finally, one evening, as he was working on the patient's chart, it suddenly hit him – this patient used 'religious' language that echoed the words of a man who had been abusive to him as a youth. His personal (and spiritual) culture rejected the religious stance he believed this patient held (based upon the man's words). Once he understood the source of his response, he was able to deal with his feelings, and thus the patient, more effectively.

Environmental factors

There are many ways to think about personal culture. Part of what determines a person's unique culture is the environment in which he was raised, or in which she currently lives. Listed below are some of the more obvious external or environmental factors that may play a role in determining who one is, and how one responds to the world and to others:

- culture
- sexual preference
- birth order
- education
- social class
- economic situation
- job
- current faith system
- family of origin
- urban/rural
- nationality.

Many of these factors are very complex, and affect us in multifaceted ways. A good example is the family of origin, which can be extremely important in terms of defining a person's personal culture. Not only do we inherit physical attributes from our parents, we inherit much more. According to one set of authors, 'we inherit a whole complex of behaviors and interactions from our families of origin.'[5] The family teaches its members how to love, how to fight, and how to use power. It teaches family members how to be alone, and how to be together with other people. All kinds of values, priorities, and even patterns of behavior are imprinted on members by the family system.

A variable that complicates the impact of family systems is birth order. The place one has within a family, their birth order position (whether first, second, last, etc.), and their sex (male or female) and the sex of the siblings can radically affect the kind of person he/she becomes.[6]

Economic status can also impact how a person thinks and functions, but it too must be looked at carefully. Economics forms people primarily through the opportunities or barriers money creates. Money can provide for education, travel, or status. It can affect where a person lives, what clothes he wears, and what kind of car he drives. It has been suggested that money, along with attractiveness and status, is one of the most powerful factors in American society.[7] Money changes things – so does a lack of money. We often hear about the 'culture of poverty' that so dramatically affects those who are raised without fiscal affluence. Without the right clothes, with little or no opportunity for an advanced (or even a basic) education, hindered by a lack of resources and tired from having to work two jobs, the person without money is clearly at a disadvantage. However, there are always exceptions. It must be remembered that there are people with great wealth and little education, and people with lots of education and little wealth. There are wealthy people who are tired and overwhelmed, and poor people who have inner peace. People go from wealth to poverty and from poverty to wealth. As with all of the facets of personal culture, when it comes to economics and its impact, each person is unique.

A factor that is often ignored, but which can have great impact, is what one author calls 'framework.'[8] A framework consists of perspectives through which an individual approaches living and believing. Each person's framework is molded fundamentally by certain key social and cultural phenomena that they experience during their formative years. The shared experiences of powerful events or phenomena, such as the depression, the death of John F Kennedy, the Vietnam War, nuclear accidents, or the explosion of the space shuttle Challenger, not only shape individuals but generations. Those who grow up together through experiences unique to their time often have a common perspective, and thus a common approach to life. They are what might be called a cohort. In his book *Frameworks*, which looks at people born between 1900 and 1972, DA Walrath identifies three basic cohorts and explores how each group is different. The three groups are the 'Strivers,' who were shaped most profoundly by the Depression, the 'Challengers,' formed by the events such as the Civil Rights Movement and Woodstock, and the 'Calculators,' who have experienced environmental deterioration, the HIV/AIDs epidemic, and the advent of terrorism.

Each of these groups sees the world differently. For the Strivers, *Stability is normal*, for the Challengers, *Change is normal*, and for the Calculators, *Erosion is normal*.

Box 5.1 Strivers (born 1900–1931)

- Strivers depend on the world continuing as it has been. The striver's life was shaped by a time of slow change. What change occurred was more development rather than transition.
- These are people with steady values.
- Their goal is *to defend our way of life*.
- They believe basic institutions are good, and are to be protected and not changed (family, nation, and church).
- Life is composed of *alternatives* to be faced. Right/wrong; good/bad; us/them. Moral behavior consists of honoring absolutes. If you work hard enough you will succeed.
- Think in terms of *oughts*.
- Lots of formulas.
- Life is duty. Satisfaction is a reward deserved by those who work hard and fulfill their obligations.
- In terms of religion they tend to focus on *morality*.

Table 5.1 Prime-time and shaping events

Birth years		Shaping years	
1900		1913	
			World War I
			Roaring Twenties
1912		1925	
	Strivers		Black Tuesday (10–29–29)
			The Depression
			The New Deal
1922		1935	
			Rise of Hitler
			Dunkirk
			Pearl Harbor
			D-Day; Holocaust
1932		1945	The Bomb
			Baby Boom
			Suburbia
1942		1955	Affluence
			Hula hoops
			Civil rights
	Challengers		JFK assassinated
1952		1965	Urban crisis (Watts riots)
			Vietnam
			RFK; MLK killed
			Woodstock
			Gas Lines
1962		1975	ERA
			Divorce
			Three Mile Island
	Calculators		Terrorism: hostage
			ERA stalled
1972		1985	Star Wars
			Shuttle explosion

Box 5.2 Challengers (born 1932–1958)

- Challengers were shaped by a period of rapid change. A disruption of old norms, values, and lifestyles. They expect life to be that way and don't even like too much stability.
- Their goal: *to alter and expand our way of life*.
- Institutions are to be examined and criticized. They want to correct ills and indulge in wants.

- They seldom see choices confined to rigid alternatives. They think in terms of *options*. Choose what you want...
- The key for this group is *wants*. They begin thinking with their own personal interests.
- This group believes you should honor your wants. They only want to work when necessary, and what work is done should be meaningful, a rewarding experience. This group feels they should be able to have it all!
- In terms of religion they tend to focus on *ethics*.

Box 5.3   Calculators (born 1959–)

- Calculators were born in a time of change, but saw some of that change as being devastating. They see change as normal, but think in terms of ever-shrinking options rather than ever-expanding options.
- Their goal: *To choose and conserve what matters most.*
- This group has never seen a time when we were not threatened by destruction (the bomb). They tend to be much more prudent and careful than the Challengers. They attempt to calculate the consequences of their decisions and choose the best possibilities left to them.
- The key to life is *consequences*.
- This group faces an ambiguous world, but is prepared to make and be confined by choices (sex and AIDS). Tomorrow's world is limited by choices made today. Sees shrinking possibilities, and seeks to protect the options chosen. They are more serious and responsible at times than even their parents.
- Think in terms of *possibilities*. However, unlike the Challengers, this group begins with the restraints.
- They will choose among options and commit themselves to what each of them sees as possible and desirable for themselves. They believe they can choose, but also that they must choose. They can't have it all!
- In terms of religion, the key word might be *piety*.

It is easy to see how these kinds of differences impact one's personal culture. These differing perspectives create different values, meanings, and even diverse approaches to spirituality.

Internal factors

People are also affected by influences that appear to be more internal. With these factors it is more a matter of who a person is, inherently or naturally, than an issue of outside forces or influences.

Some of these factors, such as gender, seem simple, but can be significantly affected by other components. With gender one is either a male or a female, a nice clean distinction. But gender can be made more complex if one adds in other factors such as sexual preference. A gay male is culturally different from a heterosexual male. Still male, but different. Add in an additional variant, such as culture, and the picture becomes even more blurred.

Other predetermined factors, such as race, are critical, but may be so broad as to provide little useful information. A person, for example, can be categorized as Hispanic, but what does that really reveal? There are Europeans who are Hispanic. There are also people who are from South America, Central America, and the Caribbean. To create a bit more focus we can add the category of nationality or geographic origin, but this still leaves a great deal of vagueness. Within Mexico, for example, there are many different ethnic groups. Ethnically this person might be a Mixteca. But even at this level we are working with a rather vague definition for there are at least 50 Mixteco dialects,[9] reflecting great diversity even among this group of about 250 000 people.[10] So we must also add to the mix the concept of culture, the unique and specific cultures to be found in specific regions, cities, or even villages. Reflecting upon this rich complexity is a powerful reminder why it is so dangerous to succumb too quickly to the allure of stereotypes.

One factor that has received a lot of attention in recent years is that of temperament. The Myers-Briggs Type Indicator (MBTI) has brought the concept of temperament or type into the mainstream of modern culture.[11] The categories of type used with the MBTI find their roots in the writings of the late Carl Jung, a Swiss psychiatrist. Jung believed that people differ in certain basic ways, even though the instincts which drive us are the same. He distinguished two general attitudes – introversion and extraversion – and four functions – thinking, feeling, sensing, and intuiting. For the purposes of this discussion what is important is the concept that each person has some inborn temperaments or types that drive their behavior, an underlying structure that is permanent and relatively unyielding. According to one author, 'people can't change form no matter how much and in what manner we require them to. Form is inherent, ingrained, indelible.'[12] If this is true, then understanding one's own type, and the type of those one interacts with, will aid in understanding and in interpersonal effectiveness. Using one of the many tools available to ascertain one's own type and to explore the type of others with whom one is in relationship is advisable for spiritual work.[13]

Another way of thinking about inherent traits is neuro-linguistics. Neruo-linguistics was pioneered by Richard Bandler and John Grinder in the 1970s. They initially explored the concept in the book *frogs into PRINCES*, published in 1979.[14] Neuro-linguistics emerged out of the observation that therapists were able to create change in their patients when they were able to identify how each patient processes information about the world.[15] The question is, how do people think? The original concept of neuro-linguistics maintained that the way people think can be captured in three broad categories, audio (words), visual (what one sees), and kinesthetic (what one feels). A more recent book on the subject adds two additional categories, olfactory (what one smells) and gustatory (what one tastes).[16] However, since we are dealing with the realm of the spirituality, we shall focus on the triumvirate of audio, visual, and kinesthetic.

Neuro-linguistics asserts that people receive and impart information through these modalities, in other words, through words, images, or feelings. Although people receive and process information through all three means, they will tend to have primary or dominant mode. If one wants to communicate effectively with a person, and connect with them in a manner that produces results, it is important to connect with them using their primary mode. When working with a person we may want to address all three modes, but we should concentrate on the primary mode of the person we are working with. How do we know? The simplest way to ascertain which mode is dominant is to listen to their language. Audio people are *word* oriented. These people are impressed with content and rational thought and are usually impressed with details and facts. They are most comfortable talking about concepts and are generally uncomfortable talking about feelings.

Box 5.4 Audio characteristics

Key words: think; idea; concept; understand; hear.
Typical phrases:

- That sounds like a good *idea*.
- I'd like to *think* about it before I answer.
- Let me *tell* you something.
- Do you *know* what I mean?
- Do you *understand* this concept?

Visual people see pictures rather than words when reading. They tend to visualize everything. They respond to visual stimulation such as art, or beauty in nature. They are often oriented toward stories.

Box 5.5 Visual characteristics

Key words: look; see; picture; vision.
Typical phrases:

- How do you *see* that event taking place?
- *Picture* it this way ...
- Can you *imagine* what it would be like?
- Let me *illustrate* it this way ...

The kinesthetic person tends to be a 'touchy feely' person. This individual is usually in touch with his/her emotions and likes to function on an emotional level.

Box 5.6 Kinesthetic characteristics

Key words: feel; emotion; touch; experience; sense.
Typical phrases:

- I was *touched* by his sincerity
- That was a *moving experience*.
- Are you with me?!

There is a need, if one is to take this aspect of personal culture seriously, to listen for the verbal clue and respond to the person in *their* mode, using their language. If you use an audio style with a kinesthetic person, chances are you will fail to communicate. Again, although all people can function in all modes, a person will tend to be most comfortable with one. We must find that one and respond in kind.

Words are not the only potential clues. One can also think in terms of body language. Think for a moment about how a person greets you. An audio person will tend to be the most reserved. With a stranger, or a casual acquaintance, the audio person might simply nod, or say 'hello' when greeting another. They may, but often will not, make any physical contact. The visual person will tend to use visual clues and will smile, look the other person in the eye, and perhaps shake the other's hand. The kinesthetic is the person most likely to touch the other physically, and do anything from shake a hand to give the other person a hug.

Imagine a patient who has come into a clinic due to chronic low back pain. What happens when the physician enters the room? The audio patient stands, nods to the physician, and says 'Hello doctor.' He puts down the pamphlet he has been reading. When asked about his chief complaint the patient responds, 'Well, I have been having a lot of trouble with my back and I *thought* it was time to get it looked at. I'm *wondering* if you can help me *understand* what is going on.' To this person the physician might reply, 'Well, let's figure out what is going on here!'

The visual patient stands, puts down the magazine he has been looking at (lots of pictures), smiles, and shakes the doctor's hand. When asked about her chief complaint she says, 'I've been having trouble with my back and it looks like I need help. I've been walking around like a little old lady, all bent over and crooked.' The physician might respond, 'Lets see if we can get a good picture of what is happening here.'

The kinesthetic person stands quickly, moves toward the physician, and shakes her hand. 'Doctor, I am so glad you are here. I am just in anguish. This back is just making me feel so depressed.' The doctor might reply. 'I'm so sorry your back is making you feel so down. I hope we can make you feel better as soon as possible.'

We can see how, in these examples, the physician moved to the dominant mode of the speaker. If we do not move to the other person's mode we may well make them nervous or uncomfortable, and we will clearly hinder the communication process. A kinesthetic response to an audio person, for example, will have the audio person backing away and feeling that their personal space has been invaded. Such a disconnect will significantly impact the therapeutic relationship.

Obviously, the task of exploring personal culture is not an easy one. There are many factors and many potential interactions between factors. This is why there are an unlimited number of variations, and why each person is best seen as a culture of one. It is clear that the complexity of personhood demands that the entire mix of factors, and the interaction of these factors with one another, must be taken into account in order to establish a relatively clear picture of an individual's personal culture.

Mental health experts may have the opportunity to explore the culture of their patients carefully. Primary care providers rarely have this luxury. In both cases, however, to whatever degree it is possible, it is best to see the process as ongoing. The goal is to take advantage of each interaction with the patient and build upon the fund of available knowledge. The healthcare professional must ask questions, listen for clues, and use those clues to ask more questions. Again, it is a process of slowly developing an understanding of this unique person with whom they are working. No one ever said developing a therapeutic relationship that addresses the whole person was easy!

Questions for reflection

- What do you believe are the key factors that impact personal culture?
- What are the most critical factors that shape *your* personal culture?
- What is your neuro-linguistic dominance? How does this impact how you give and receive information?
- Write a description of yourself. Be creative (one described themselves using the format of a birdbook).
- What are the 'points of intensity'? What aspects of your personal culture are most likely to aid or hinder your work with others?

Spiritual cultures

Obviously, if we are going to work with a person around spiritual issues we must think specifically about a person's spiritual culture. Each person also has a spiritual culture that is the result of the interface between their personal culture and the spiritual experiences or frameworks to which they have been exposed. A person's spiritual culture can include such components as religious affiliation or prefer- ence, spiritual practices – both traditional and non-traditional – past spiritual experiences, and his/her unique spiritual thinking. In terms of spiritual culture there seem to be three major groups of people. The first group is those people who have an active connection with a specific religion and a specific community of faith. The second group is made up of those people who are not currently involved in a community of faith, but have a 'religious' background that is important to them or has significantly impacted their current spiritual culture. The third group includes those people whose spiritual lives have been impacted lightly, or not at all, by major faith systems and specific communities of faith. Although our approach to inte- gration will demand that we approach all people essentially the same way, which group people belong to may affect or guide the focus of our interactions, and in some cases the 'language' of our interactions. Let us begin by looking at each of these groups in more detail.

For those who participate in a community of faith this organized spiritual entity may well be the most important factor for understanding their spiritual cultures and their perspectives about illness and healing. However, when talking to a person who participates in a particular religious system, it is not necessary to have a comprehensive knowledge of that system in order be effective. The idea that one must become a 'theologian' in order to work with people around spiritual issues is a barrier that keeps healthcare professionals from addressing the spiritual realm.[17] This fear can be circumvented if we think about the goals related to the integration of spirituality and medicine. Our goals are to address spiritual issues that are obstacles to healing and to access spiritual resources that facilitate healing. Thus, what we truly need to understand is how a person sees their spirituality and their illness interfacing. How do their spiritual beliefs affect the perceived meaning or value of their illness? How do their beliefs affect their outlook; do they make them hopeful, or induce a sense of dread? Are there components to their faith system that can be used to support the healing process? In short, those particular beliefs that address illness, healing, and death are most important.

There are resources that provide some information about the basic health beliefs of major religions. In its chapter on Cultural Awareness, for example, *Mosby's Guide to Physical Examination* provides an outstanding table on 'Religious Beliefs That Affect Patient Care.'[18] Mosby's focuses on beliefs about birth and death, diet and food practices, and about medical care (healing). It also adds a few comments that help the reader understand some of the unique aspects of the religion, either in terms of attitudes or beliefs, or in terms of faith practices. It would be useful for practitioners to review these kinds of general summaries in order to build a foundation for understanding the perspectives of their patients.[19]

Unfortunately such overviews are very limited in their applicability and it must be recognized that within each religion there is a diversity of belief and teaching which occurs at almost all levels. One can find radically different beliefs within religions, denominations (subgroups within religions), and even within individual faith communities. To make matters more convoluted, when we take a particular faith perspective, such as Baha'i, Hinduism, Buddhism, Christian, Islam, or Judaism, and combine that spiritual culture with the personal culture of the individual, an even more unique perspective emerges. A Christian Presbyterian from a rural area may be quite different from a Christian Presbyterian from an urban area, the differences of their individual churches aside. A person who has lost people close to him through death may have a perspective quite different from a person in the same church who has not experienced such a loss. A person who has had significant health issues may have a spiritual perspective about illness that is very distinct from a person who has never been seriously ill. Yet for all of its limitation, religious preference is still a good place to start with many people as it will deeply impact their views about illness, death, and healing.

There are, of course, many people who do not practice their spirituality in the context of a community of faith, but instead practice it in very individualistic and personal ways. But this does not mean that we should not explore the idea of religious preference with this group as well. We should never underestimate the significance of religion in people's lives, even if they are not currently involved in a church, synagogue, or other religious community. In America over 60% of the people believe religion is very important, and only 12% believe it is 'not very important.'[20] This is not just an American phenomenon. A poll conducted in 1996 in India showed 59% of the populace defining themselves as 'very religious' and only 6% identifying themselves as 'not very religious.' In spite of the fact that there is a perception that religious groups are declining in popularity, that far fewer people are participating in community worship, and that the influence of religious groups on the culture is declining, the place of religion remains relatively stable. The fact is that between 1938 and 1998 the percentage of people who happened 'to attend church or synagogue in the last seven days' remained constant. In 1938, 41% answered in the affirmative, compared to 40% in 1998.[21] When asked about religious preference, 94% of Americans named a preference (Protestant, Catholic, Jewish, Muslim, Hindu, Buddhist, etc.) while only 6% did not identify a prefer-ence.[22] Far more people claim religious preference than claim religious member-ship. This is true for several reasons. First, faith groups vary greatly on their standards for membership and in some cases people attend regularly but are not considered 'members.' Second, many people clearly identify with a church even if they do not participate actively in a specific community of faith.

Even among those people who practice their spirituality in non-traditional ways there is often an underlying historical connection with a particular faith system. Thus it is important when talking to people who do not currently participate in a community of faith, to ascertain whether they participated in a community of faith earlier in life, or whether they identify with a particular faith system. If they have a connection, that background will often have a significant effect on their spiritual culture. Sometimes the impact of an earlier exposure to a faith system will be formative in the positive sense. Many of the beliefs and values which were imparted by the faith of childhood will remain integrated into a person's personal system. In other cases this exposure may be essentially negative, driving the person to a spiritual stance that is in contrast to what was taught by that original faith system.

When working with people who have a current religious connection and with those who are not active in a faith community, but can articulate a religious preference or even historical relationship with a faith system, the main focus must remain on how their religious context or background affects the way they think about illness, death, and healing. Because of their belief system, what meaning does their illness have for them? Is it just something that happens? Is it something 'allowed' by God to get their attention? Is it something 'caused' by God to teach them a lesson, or punish them? What role does the sacred, the church, the spiritual aspect of one's being have in the process of healing? It is also important to explore the progress of their faith. It is not just where they are currently, but how they got there. Where did they start? How is their current set of beliefs and values the same or different from where they began? If there is a difference in belief, what is that difference and what was the catalyst for change?

Although we must take seriously the importance of earlier faith experiences, we must also remember that many people (44% of Americans) are 'not religious' and have not participated in the activities of a community of faith in the previous six months.[23] There is a great variance from country to country, and even from region to region within countries on this issue. In the American South the prevailing culture is religious, with a relatively high percentage (61%) of people participating in communities of faith, and religion having a powerful influence on regional culture. In the American West this influence is greatly muted, with only 48% of the populace being involved in communities of faith. Indeed the Northwest has high percentages of people who consider themselves 'non-religious.' In one study 21% of Oregonians, 25% of Washingtonians, and 19% of those in Idaho said they had 'no religion.'[24] This can be contrasted with 11% of Texans, 6% of those in Alabama, and 7% in Mississippi. But non-religious does not necessarily mean non-spiritual. Remember, 'almost two-thirds of Americans confidently affirm God's existence. Ninety-five percent of the American public believe in God or what they term a "High Power." '[25] When talking with those who are spiritual but have no clear connection with a faith system, the focus will be different. Instead of looking at the community of faith one will look at personal faith practices. Formal worship will probably become unimportant, but personal practices such as meditation and prayer may become more important. Beliefs about healing will not be community centered, but individually centered. Images of the sacred or divine will become more diverse. The focus will become less doctrinal and more experiential. Since most people live in larger 'cultures' that tend to be heavily influenced by a dominant religion, there will likely be some influence exerted by that religion. However, it will be 'second hand' and will truly be 'cultural' rather than informed and intentional.

Questions for reflection

- What are your spiritual 'roots'?
- In what ways has your spiritual heritage shaped you?
- What is your current spiritual framework or culture?

What is critical is that interactions with others around spirituality and health truly be an exploration of the individual's personal culture. The temptation is to do what is easy, place a religious 'tag' on the person and assume that tells us enough. But we cannot take what we know about religious or faith systems and try and make people fit into those models. We must do the hard work. Yes, it is hard work. Yes, it takes time. Yes, it is a process. No, it doesn't fit easily into the model of a 15-minute appointment. But it can be done. In the context of an ongoing therapeutic relationship the process of listening, gathering information, and learning to appreciate the complexity of a person's spiritual thinking can take place. We can help those we interact with to construct, or perhaps reconstruct, their spiritual framework – and then apply it to their illness. For some the process will go quickly, for they will be people who have thought about what their illness means and how it fits into the larger picture. They will be able to identify ways in which their spiritual thinking might be creating issues for them, contributing to a sense of dis-ease and perhaps playing a causal role with respect to their disease.

For others it will take more time. Some patients will not have a clue what is going on within them spiritually. It will be happening, but awareness will be missing. At times they will have vague understanding, but will not be able to connect the dots. This group will need to be coached about how to think spiritually. They will need to expand their understanding of their spiritual framework and be able to identify the positive and negative aspects of their spiritual culture. They will need to recognize how their spiritual health is affecting their physical health, and think about what spiritual resources can be applied to the healing process. With this group the process may move slowly. That's alright! Just as physical issues cannot always be 'fixed' or even identified quickly, so sometimes spiritual issues find resolution only over time.

The task of those in the 'healing' role is not, again, to be a spiritual expert. It is primarily to play a facilitative role, to help generate spiritual discovery, understanding, growth, and resolution as part of the process of healing. When we fulfill this role we will find that patients will be able to make both a journey inward and a journey outward. They will be able to go into the depths of their person, and explore all aspects of who they are, including their spirituality. Then they will be able to express that spirituality and apply it to their life and their illness. As the process unfolds, and as people begin to share their spiritual thinking, what we will hear will be unique and powerful. Sometimes it will be joyful and empowering, at other times disturbing. Hopefully it will always be helpful.

Personal spirituality

In 2004 we took some time to explore the way a diverse group of people thought spiritually about illness, health, healing, and death. A questionnaire was sent to around 80 people who were both patients and healthcare professionals. Those who participated were from a number of countries and many spiritual systems. Some were part of organized religions, others were not. Their responses illustrate powerfully the kind of unique and helpful information that can emerge when we take the time to look at unique spiritual cultures. We started by exploring the concept of spirituality itself, for how one thinks about spirituality heavily influences how one thinks about illness, health, and healing. A key question on the questionnaire that was sent to 100 people across the United States and in several foreign countries was 'Please describe your personal spirituality.' The first thing that becomes clear in looking at the responses is that there are many unique ways to think about spirituality, even among people from essentially the same faith system. Following are some of the responses, clustered by faith system.

Muslim

> Spirituality to me is something inside me that keeps me going rather than anything connected to religion. I believe that every person has a spirit that lives with him/her, and I also believe that the spirit is connected to the rest of the world at a totally different level.
>
> Jamal, 34

> In spite of the fact that outgoing from the philosophy of Kant, I consider that it is impossible to demonstrate either existence of God, or his non-existence through science, I am a believer in the sense that the world without God for me is boring and intolerable. God and religion for me are the basis of activating, energizing of my spiritual nature.
>
> Mehdi, 53

> Spirituality is an integral part of life. This is something that should guide any person throughout his or her life. I believe that this is the concept of my religion, which guides you in any case and condition of one's life, and the objective of a person should be to abide to the principles of Islam.
>
> Elshad, 30

These three men are all from the same general geographic area, Baku, Azerbaijan. One is involved in non-profit work, one is a scientist, and the other is a physician. All of them were raised when Azerbaijan was part of the United Soviet Socialist Republic (USSR) and were raised in an environment where Islam was more cultural than religious. Two of them, Mehdi and Elshad, have had a 'religious awakening' and have become 'active' in the practice of Islam. Jamal still considers his ties to Islam more ethnic or cultural. All three have a unique perspective of spirituality. For Jamal spirituality is real, but very personal and more a matter of inner energy or power. When asked about spiritual practices, he was unable to identify one. For Elshad spirituality is clearly defined by his religion, and by the rules put forth by that religion through its scriptures and traditions. When asked about spiritual practices he talks about the 'five main requirements of Islam' and describes clearly a set of religious disciplines Those disciplines are:

1 **Shahadat:** testifying that there is no other God than Allah and Mohammad is his messenger
2 **Namaz:** praying five times a day
3 **Oruj:** fasting during the month of Ramadan
4 **Zakat:** sharing part of your property with people around you
5 **Haj:** pilgrimage to Mecca.

For Mehdi also, faith is strongly shaped by his religion, but he sees faith less in terms of 'following the rules' and more in terms of spiritual energy. Although he has spiritual practices they are more individual and unique. They include prayer, reading, and reading the Koran, similar to Elshad, but also include reading the Torah, the Christian Bible, and other 'divine books.'

Their ideas about illness and healing reflect the uniqueness of their personal faith cultures. Having different faith frameworks they endow illness with different meanings, and think about healing in diverse ways.

> It is possible that an illness is not just God's punishment, but God's ordeal and sign (omen).
>
> Mehdi

> Whatever happens is the will of God... Islam accepts the concept of being ill and getting cured, but treatment itself should be found in purification of both body and soul... First of all Islam stands for taking care of body as the body itself is not yours and it is rented to you for use, custody, and care... Sunah regulate the behavior and actions of a person, and all of the requirements, at deeper analysis, prove to serve the healthy lifestyle... [translation: illness comes from not following the religious rules leading to a healthy lifestyle]
>
> Elshad

> I think illness is caused by the disruption of balance in the energy of the person. In other words, it might be a lack of energy to fight the illness at any given time. Illness might also be caused by the lack of belief that one can overcome this illness, which essentially causes the lack of energy to struggle with it.
>
> Jamal

As we can see from these three responses, these men theologize about illness in very different ways. For two there is a sense that illness has something to do with the will of Allah, but one clearly adds the element of personal responsibility. Ignore the health rules set down by God and you will get sick. For the third, illness has to do with a lack of energy, by a person being 'out of balance.'

It is not surprising therefore, to find some interesting diversity when they begin to think about healing. For Jamal, healing is very much a spiritual exercise (although he cannot identify any 'religious' component to healing or name any 'practices' that aid cure). 'Cure has either a purely medical base, or it could be done through acquiring some positive energy.' For Elshad, healing comes in part by following the 'rules' set up by the Quran and the Sunahs. As one actively lives one's faith, and 'purifies both body and soul' cure is possible. Mehdi, perhaps showing the influence of other faith systems on his spiritual culture, says, 'I think, that really prayer can cure the person. I repeatedly have experienced it. The prayer will mobilize, will actuate spiritual energy of the person in a direction of his/her illness.'

We offer these three men as examples because their stories illustrate well the concept of a 'culture of one,' and the way individual spiritual cultures emerge. In the case of these men, integrating spirituality into the healing process would look very different for each one of them. For Jamal the focus might well be on the development of spiritual energy. For Mehdi the focus might be on prayer, within the context of his religious practices. For Elshad discussions might center on spiritual purity and life practices. We have not in any way moved to a level of great depth through the survey, but even at this entry level we find concepts expressed that can be explored and used as part of the therapeutic process.

Roman Catholic

We see a similar diversity of thought among a group of Roman Catholic respondents. Again, the wide range of views about spirituality causes this group to create diverse meanings about illness, and unique ideas about the role of spirituality in healing.

> *My personal spirituality* is 'giving funds to organizations.'
> *Illness* 'happens because there are germs in the air, crazy drivers, etc.'
> *Healing or cure* is 'in God's hands, whether we live or die – and a good doctor is a vital asset.'
>
> Anonymous, 74, USA

> *My personal spirituality* is 'a synthesis of Ignatian and Benedictine/ Cistercian spiritualities.'
> *Illness* 'is part of our common humanity, our human nature.'
> *Healing or cure* is 'reconciliation with our selves, those we love, and with God.'
>
> Tim, 44, USA

> *My personal spirituality* is 'not a defined religion, but a sense of God in nature ... connectedness of the natural world.'
> *Illness* 'in many cases is the result of personal lifestyle choices, sometimes it is genetic... I feel there is more of a mystery concerning how and why individuals succumb to illness... It's illogical but while I do not believe that God causes illness, God may play a part in good health or recovery.'
> *Healing or cure*: 'I think rather pragmatically. By rallying round the troops /gathering all opportunities for healing/cure via medical science, combining it with support systems, faith, and personal responsibility for recovery, optimistically the outcome will be positive. If not, acceptance.'
>
> Karen, 49, USA

> *My personal spirituality:* I strongly believe that a person's faith is something that is very personal and should not be worn on their shirt sleeve. Each of us serves as a judge of our own faith and should be satisfied with our own status with God before trying to judge that of others.
> *Illness:* While the onset of many illnesses can be traced directly to one's personal choices, I believe that a significant portion of it is bound to happen regardless of our actions or choices. A part of staying healthy is

taking timely preventative measures to find major problems at their earliest onset rather than procrastinating in spite of evidence that something needs to be done. From my perspective, denial in the face of evidence is more prevalent in my father's generation than mine but is still a significant issue for Irish Catholic males. So, while I do not believe that God necessarily causes illness, I do believe that each of us live in a world between hypochondria and absolute denial that is largely shaped by our culture.

Healing or cure: Taking personal responsibility for ones own health is the first step to staying healthy. Those who do not take responsibility do not tend to heal as quickly or completely as those who have an investment in staying healthy and getting healthy.

Kevin, 53, USA

The diversity expressed by this group is not without significance. For our Catholic who clearly sees spirituality as 'doing good things,' the role of spirituality in healing is simple – prayer. In terms of spiritual practices – 'just obey the doctor's orders.' Tim, a theologically sophisticated Catholic, sees spirituality as 'a constant resource, reminder, and anchor of "seeing God in all things."' Spirituality connects us with the divine and thus with a power for healing and good. There is no specific healing ritual for Tim, but there is the need for 'an ongoing awareness to be present to the "sacrament of the present moment."' Karen, who is in the process of moving spiritually out of her Roman Catholic roots to a broader non-denominational stance, is not sure about the role of spirituality in healing. 'My belief is currently that a deity exists but is rather hands-off. Spirituality consistent with that is for an individual to make every personal effort to recover, combining the science of medicine with whatever support their faith affords.' She adopts a stance common to many American Christians, that healing is a cooperative effort between the individual, the medical professional, and the divine. However, with her the weight of responsibility remains with the individual to work toward recovery. Again, there are no healing practices or rituals beyond 'typical de-stressing and health recovery practices such as nature walks and exercise.' Kevin, a product of a rural area and an Irish Catholic culture, focuses on a very private faith and on personal responsibility.

Again what it is important to recognize is that each person has developed their own unique beliefs about spirituality, the meaning of illness, the nature of healing, and the role of spirituality in healing. It is this unique perspective we must capture if we are to engage a person's spirituality in the process of healing. The point is that there are as many spiritual cultures or perspectives as there are people. Each person has a definition of spirituality that is unique. Each person finds a value or meaning in illness that is distinctive. The first task of integration is to help people explore, discover, and articulate their spiritual culture. Only then can we move on toward functional integration.

Following are some selected comments from other people, each a reflection of the rich diversity that can be found in those around us. In this plurality of views are present wonderful resources that can aid the process of healing. Also present may be barriers that hinder recovery. Either way, these unique spiritual perspectives are illustrative of the powerful viewpoints that shape the way people respond to illness and engage in the process of healing.

'I believe in faith very strongly and view religion as a form to define faith and to use that as a modem for spiritual wellbeing... I attend temple gatherings periodically, pray every day using the traditional Hindu offerings, read the Bagavad Gita periodically... Genetics and environment have a strong role in the cause of illness and it is faith that sustains us through the illness. Faith also defines how we react toward illness and plays a pivotal role in our healing process...

Sumanthi, 36, Hindu, India

I was born in atheist family and become religious at 29 years of age. My religion is Armenian Apostolic Church. I reflect much about God and his role in my life... Disease comes from whole mode of life, work, food, and heredity... in certain conditions perhaps the cause is God... When people believe in God he lightly transfer her disease... God helps people mobilize all reserves...

Narine, 42, Christian, Armenia

I believe spirituality has all to do with developing positive attributes... I follow Eknath Easwaran's eight-point program ... I believe that science and religion go hand in hand. Some illness is caused by germs – some by accidents, some by genetics – whatever. I believe there exists physical, emotional, psychological, and spiritual illnesses. Perhaps there are two kinds of ordeals, one to test the soul ... and one is 'karma' for our actions... I believe there are two kinds of healing, material means and spiritual means... I believe that all true healing comes from God and through the power of the Holy Spirit. I also believe the ultimate outcome is totally the Will of God... I do not believe that prevailing diseases are related to our sins. I do believe that disease can remind us of the temporary nature of earthly life... I pray for those who are ill, I visit them, and in certain cases, I use therapeutic touch...

Jeanne, 61, Baha'i, USA

Spirituality, in the sense of meaning and purpose, affects what I do in relationships... Illness happens. Some is preventable by better health habits. Illness can teach us something if we are of the mindset to learn. It can help us be empathetic to others experiencing illness... The Bible presents anointing as a way of asking for healing. Healing outside of traditional medical cures can happen. I don't think God generally intervenes this way. He is not in the job of reversing consequences of our negative choices... I don't think healing is related to the amount of faith one has. It is God's decision. Our spirituality could be such that although our body may not heal, our spirit is whole in God.

Nancy, 61, Seventh Day Adventist, USA

My spirituality is humanist mixed with Judeo-Christian and some Far Eastern religious beliefs ... Initially (when sick) I ask if there is something I did or didn't do – absolutely *not* God-caused, believe in some randomness ... I believe there is healing power in positive value-based actions/thoughts ... does not mean cure, more a state of being that one is OK, in tune with values and doing the right thing no matter what the outcomes physically.

Gary, age NA, Unitarian-Universalist, USA

I am a liberal Christian, a big follower of William Sloan Coffin. Illness can flow out of lifestyle, but cancer is not caused by anything, just the way life is ... need solid spiritual background in order to make lifestyle changes that are required in illness ... need social support, strong belief in self, etc. ... God is in everything.

Kiame, 25, Lutheran, Republic of Congo

My personal spirituality entails a belief in the power of positive and negative human energy and activity to generate galvanizing effects in oneself, another individual, or in small or large groups of people... I understand illness in many different ways, including: genetic misfortune, adaptive and maladaptive biological adjustments to internal and external change (including aging), and learned behavioral responses to interpersonal and environmental stressors. I do not envision Higher Power causation for illness. Similarly, illness can be imbued with many meanings, including the gift of humility, as contrast for better appreciation of one's health, as warning to slow down or improve health habits and self-care, as catalyst for acknowledging one's vulnerability, frailty, and mortality, and as rehearsal for aging and dying... I view healing as the process of becoming as whole and healthy as one is capable of becoming in a given situation and a particular stage of life, given one's endowments, encumbrances, and past history. I'm not sure if I believe in the notion of cure as conventionally defined (return to prior state of health following the resolution or eradication of an illness or disease). I think what is often called a cure is really more like arriving at a new unique state of health that is hard to compare with one's 'pre-morbid' state ... fashion. I hold open the possibility of some kind of Higher Power energy contributing to healing or cure.

Michael, 58, Unitarian-Universalist, USA

I believe in being conscious and aware, in knowing what is unknowable, out of reach of our awareness (to this I put any specifics about God, if there is one, and calls into doubt most spiritual epiphanies). To some extent I suppose this belief in ... nothing ... could be a certain spiritual belief... but often one that often comes into direct conflict with organized spiritual activities... I try not to [think about illness or cure]... I believe that an important element in healing is the relationship that the patient has with others, with themselves, with their doctor, with their beliefs such as God and religion.

Joshua, 39, no religion, USA

Bad stuff happens to good people. We have some power to take control of our bodies and our spiritual and mental lives in preventing accidents, illness, etc.... Personal attitudes are very important in how we heal... I see the spiritual as the power of health and goodness, sometimes fighting off darker forces – I guess I'm Manichean.

Rich, 62, agnostic, USA

When a free and friendly space is created people will begin to share who they really are. Not only will they begin to reveal their own personal cultures, which are rich and varied, but they will also, often cautiously, begin to share their spiritual framework. What is being offered here is a great gift, that of the self. And through this gift the possibility for an entirely new kind of therapeutic relationship emerges – a healing partnership that addresses not just the physical body, but the entire person. It is important that we remember the basic principles we have established First, that each person is a culture of one. Second, that if we are to be able to understand another's unique culture, and the forces that have shaped and continue to shape them, we must understand our own unique culture. Third, that if we would move with people into the realm of the spiritual, we must understand that each person also has a unique set of spiritual beliefs or values. Fourth, if we would discover people's unique spiritual values, we must learn how to communicate, learn how to receive and send messages in such a way that we move through the shallowness to the core feelings and beliefs within.

As we move forward the next task will be to look at some of the tools we can use for exploring the spiritual culture. This will provide the basis for the integrated encounter. From this initial therapeutic act it will then be necessary to take two additional steps. First we will need to learn how to think about what we have discovered, in short we will need to think about the spiritual dynamics present in the other, and make some sort of assessment. It is this assessment that will provide the foundation for the next step, intervention. Having exposed spiritual dynamics it is important to support and access the spiritual strengths revealed and/or address the spiritual issues that may be hindering the work of healing. The integration of spiritual and healthcare means working together to make things happen! A final issue is that of continuity. How do we continue to walk with people, through health, illness, healing, and through life itself?

Questions for reflection

- Please describe your personal spirituality.
- What are your personal spiritual practices (prayer, bible reading, Torah, meditation, other reading, group experiences, etc.)
- How do you think (or theologize) about illness? In other words, what is the meaning or value of illness for you?
- How to you think (theologize) about healing or cure?
- How do you view the role of God/divine/sacred in terms of healing or cure?
- What is the role of your spirituality in terms of healing or cure?
- Does your spiritual perspective include any healing rituals or practices?

Notes

1   Mehrabian A (1971) *Silent Messages*. Wadsworth, Belmont, CA.
2   The communication models used in this section are based on models developed by John L Wallen and included in the Lab I: Skills for Calling and Caring Ministries, 'Learning the Language of Healing,' published by LEAD Consultants, Inc., Reynoldsburg, OH, 1982.
3   McKay M, Davis M and Fanning P (1983) *Messages: the communication book*. New Harbinger Publications, Oakland, CA.

4   McKay M, Davis M and Fanning P (1983) *Messages: the communication book*. New Harbinger Publications, Oakland, CA, p.8.

5   Roman M and Raley P (1980) *The Indelible Family*. Rawson, Wade Publishers, New York, NY, p.15.

6   Richardson R and Richardson L (1990) *Birth Order and You*. Self-Counsel Press, Bellingham, WA. (This is one example of the many books available to explore this factor. This one is easy to access and has a very practical focus.)

7   Foster R (1985) *Money, Sex and Power*. Harper, San Francisco, CA.

8   Walrath DA (1987) *Frameworks: patterns for living and believing today*. The Pilgrim Press, New York, NY.

9   Listing of current dialects can be found at www.ethnologue.com/show_country. asp?name=Mexico.

10 Brief description of the Mixteca people can be found at www.newadvent.org/cathen/ 10409a.htm.

11 Myers I (1962) *Manual: the Myers-Briggs Type Indicator*. Consulting Psychologists Press, Palo Alto, CA.

12 Keirsey D and Bates M (1984) *Please Understand Me*. Prometheus Nemesis Books, Del Mar, CA, p.2.

13 A popular tool that provides a simplified type analysis is Keirsey and Bates' book *Please Understand Me*. Other books look not only at type, but apply them to marriage relationship, work, and even the church. The Alban Institute, for example, created a book *Personality Type and Religious Leadership*. The goal of this book, which provides a very crude tool for identifying one's type, is to look at the implication of type for pastoral leadership. Oswald R and Kroeger O (1988) *Personality Type and Religious Leadership*. Alban Institute, Washington, DC. Another book, focusing on types and spirituality, is Hirsh SK and Kise JAG (1998) *Soul Types*. Hyperion Press, New York, NY.

14 Bandler R and Grinder J (1979) *frogs into PRINCES*. Real People Press, Moab, UT.

15 Bandler R and Grinder J (1979) *frogs into PRINCES*. Real People Press, Moab, UT, p.10.

16 Walker L (2002) *Consulting with NLP: neuro-linguistic programming in the medical consultation*. Radcliffe Medical Press, Oxford.

17 Ellis M, Vinson D and Ewigman B (1999) Addressing spiritual concerns with patients: family physician attitudes and practices. *Journal of Family Practice*. **48**(2): 105–9.

18 Seidel HM, Ball JW, Dains JE and Benedict GW (1995) *Mosby's Guide to Physical Examination* (3e). Mosby, St Louis, MO, pp.40–5 (Table 2–2).

19 See appendix for the Pediatric Nursing overview.

20 Gallup G Jr and Lindsay MD (1999) *Surveying the Religious Landscape*. Morehouse Publishing, Harrisburg, PA, p.10.

21 Gallup G Jr and Lindsay MD (1999) *Surveying the Religious Landscape*. Morehouse Publishing, Harrisburg, PA, p.15.

22 Gallup G Jr and Lindsay MD (1999) *Surveying the Religious Landscape*. Morehouse Publishing, Harrisburg, PA, p.16.

23 Gallup G Jr and Lindsay MD (1999) *Surveying the Religious Landscape*. Morehouse Publishing, Harrisburg, PA, p.96.

24 Source: American Religious Identification Survey by the Graduate Center of the City University of New York. Found at www.usatoday.com/graphics/news/gra/ gnoreligion/flash.htm.

25 Gallup G Jr and Lindsay MD (1999) *Surveying the Religious Landscape*. Morehouse Publishing, Harrisburg, PA, p.23.

CHAPTER 6

The objectives of integrating spirituality and medicine

> Teachers can only be teachers when there are students who want to be students. Without a question, an answer is experience as manipulation; without a struggle, help is considered interference; and without a desire to learn, the offer to teach is easily felt as oppression. Therefore, our first task is not to offer information, advice, or even guidance, but to allow others to come into touch with their own struggles, pains, doubts, and insecurities – in short, to affirm their life as quest.
>
> Henri Nouwen, *Seeds of Hope*[1]

In Chapter 2 we explored the reluctance of many physicians to integrate spirituality into practice.[2] Among the major concerns voiced by providers is a lack of clarity about the goals of integration. That concern, voiced by almost half the respondents in one survey, reflects 'uncertainty about how to manage spiritual issues raised by patients.'[3] This can be restated through the following questions.

- If I uncover spiritual issues in patients, what do I do with them?
- Should I initiate an intervention?
- If I intervene, what am I trying to accomplish?
- Are spiritual issues beyond the scope of healthcare? Is this my job?

Recognizing that people have unique personal and spiritual cultures, and believing that those cultures can impact the process of healing either positively or negatively, how do we respond? Clearly this depends on what we want to accomplish. It is probably safe to say that the ultimate reason for addressing spiritual issues in the healthcare context should be healing. By addressing not only a person's physical issues, but also their relational, emotional, and spiritual ones, clinicians can help patients find relief from not only disease but also dis-ease, and address the total state of illness. In short, they can help create spiritual change and growth, or support a spirituality that aids the process of healing. But what are the core objectives we need to achieve in order to reach that goal? If we understand these objectives, then we will be able to establish appropriate methodology for integrating spirituality into the healthcare context.

A recent survey of hospital chaplains established a list of desired outcomes for spiritual counseling in the healthcare setting. Those outcomes are as follows.[4]

- Give the client something to think about.
- Help identify key stressors.
- Restore hope/faith/harmony.
- Help deal with ambiguity.
- Renew purpose/meaning.

- Provide closure.
- Help resolve issues identified.

This list provides us with an excellent sense of the purpose of intervention. Much of what is reflected in these proposed objectives is what might be called 'self-awareness' – awareness not only of needs, but also of values and goals. These objectives also present the concept that there may need to be evolution in the way the person thinks. A shift, for example, from despair to hope or from anger to forgiveness. Also reflected in these objectives is the concept of change or resolution. Sometimes the act of changing the way one perceives or thinks about life or illness is a critical change in itself. But there are often other changes that need to occur. A clinical encounter can become a time to explore, however briefly, spiritual options. Finally, these objectives include the concept of nurture or support. The entire process must take place in an atmosphere of trust and compassion. Indeed, without the proper relational environment, integration of spiritual care with healthcare is unlikely to occur at any meaningful level. It is possible to organize the objectives of spiritual intervention into the following broad categories:

- self-awareness
- amplification
- reframing
- creation of options
- empathy and support.

In establishing these objectives, the context must clearly be taken into account. The primary purpose of the medical encounter is physical health. Many physicians believe that all other agendas must be submissive to this primary agenda. While most medical providers receive some training in how to deal with psychosocial issues and, increasingly, spiritual issues,[5] this is not their area of primary expertise and there are limits to how they might respond to spiritual distress. Finally, there is the issue of time. In the survey conducted by Mark Ellis, Daniel C Vinson, and Bernard Ewigman, time was the most commonly mentioned barrier, at 71%, to the integration of medicine and spirituality.[6] So whatever is accomplished must happen within this framework of multiple agendas, limited expertise, and minimal time.

Self-awareness

When feelings are strong, communication is often indirect. Issues and struggles are contained in stories, body language, tone of voice, and indirect expressions of feeling. In some cases this camouflage is related to the issue of trust. When we express deep and powerful feelings it makes us vulnerable. When another person knows how we feel, they have a certain power over us. Anthony Campolo, a professor of sociology, reflects this reality in what he calls the 'principle of least interest,'[7] which asserts that the person who loves the most has the least power. In other words, the person who is the most open, and gives the most emotionally, is the most vulnerable. Thus we often reveal ourselves cautiously and progressively. The more trust grows, the more we are able to reveal.

However, in many other instances the feelings and issues we reveal are vague and cloaked primarily because we are at least to some degree unaware of our own feelings and struggles. We are out of touch with ourselves, and thus are unable to understand and resolve our issues. This is why the definition of psychopathology for most models of psychotherapy includes the concept that people are essentially cut off from various aspects of their selves. Freud, for example, argued that the main purpose of therapy was to make the unconscious conscious. For him the goal of therapy was to help the individual become aware of all the feelings, motivations, and impulses that had been forgotten or repressed.[8] Carl Jung also believed the goal of psychotherapy was to help people become aware of ideas from the unconscious of which they were formerly unaware.[9] Carl Rogers, the phenomenologist, although not focused on the unaware, does stress the importance of people being open to all their thoughts and feelings. When people are not open, it is normally due to a belief that those feelings are somehow unacceptable and thus must be denied or ignored.[10] In general, when one looks at psychological models through the years, one theme is dominant: awareness of the self is important, whether it be the exposure of what was unconscious or clarification of conscious thoughts and perceptions.

It is difficult for people to work on and resolve issues of which they are unaware. A person who does not recognize the presence of anger is unlikely to move toward forgiveness. A sense of helplessness, unobserved, will remain not only hidden, but pervasive. If people are to grow, if they are to move toward authenticity and reach their potential, then they must identify those feelings and issues that control them. Otherwise those feelings and issues imprison and ultimately define and them.

Al is a 39-year-old Hispanic male. For years Al has struggled with a number of health issues, including obesity and diabetes. Al has tried a variety of treatment plans, most of which have had initial success. But each time Al starts losing significant amounts of weight or appears to get his blood glucose under control, he suddenly changes his behavior, effectively sabotaging his efforts. This self-defeating behavior has also carried over into other areas of his life. He has obtained a series of jobs, but each time he appears to be settling in, several times even on the verge of promotion, he engages in behavior that results in his being fired.

During one primary care visit, his physician used a behavior description with Al. He described Al's pattern of moving toward success, both in terms of his medical condition and his life, and his disruption of that success. His purpose was simple: to ask Al why this pattern existed. Much to his surprise, Al was totally shocked by the description of his behavior. He had been in denial and had refused to recognize this pattern in himself.

'Wow!' he responded, 'I really do that don't I! Why?'

The physician simply repeated the query.

'That is a good question, why do you think this happens?'

After a relatively brief conversation Al concluded, 'I'm afraid to succeed. I know I'm not very smart. If I succeed then I'll be asked to do something I can't do, and I'll fail. It is better to fail on purpose.'

The doctor continued to ask questions.

'But how does that relate to your health? How can you fail there?'

'I'm comfortable,' Al responded, 'as a fat dumb guy. That's who I am. If I am successful, if I lose weight, then things change. I guess I'm afraid.'

'Afraid?' responded the physician.

'No, that's not right,' said Al.

'I've done some really bad things in my life. I'm comfortable with being fat, and being sick, 'cause it fits, you know, my being bad. It's what I deserve. It's like God smackin' me.'

'Let's talk about that for a moment,' counters the provider.

One psychologist describes self-awareness as 'the process of examining oneself in the mirror.'[11] It is a matter of seeing one's behavior, perceptions, or feelings in a clear way.

When self-awareness emerges, people begin to understand the forces that shape them, control them. They begin to get in touch with what might be called 'life commandments,' those rules that guide the way they think and act. They start to understand their beliefs and values, about God, their illness, and life in general. Al, in the previous case study, began to understand his basic belief in his own 'badness' and how that belief was affecting his health and life.

Sometimes what is learned provides the foundation for recovery. As people work with their provider, they find, deep within themselves, empowering spiritual beliefs such as a belief in their inherent value as a person and a positive meaning for their current distress. This positive awareness may make the difference between a person coping with an illness, or becoming defeated by it. It may move them forward and allow positive actions.

On the other hand, what emerges may be negative, patterns of belief that inhibit recovery. This too is a positive development. Although such awareness may be painful, it is ultimately enabling. As one clinician notes:

> ...one might prefer to put a Band-Aid on an infected wound. However, it is generally better, though more painful, to clean out the wound first before applying a dressing. The same idea is to be applied to our internal thoughts and images ... before negative thoughts and images can be dealt with and modified, the individual must be made aware of them and have a grasp of their central content.[12]

The bottom line is that self-awareness provides patients and clinicians with the raw material necessary for healing. When there is awareness, strengths can be applied to the process of dealing with disease or dis-ease, and people can begin to address those issues that are hindering them from moving forward. In short, awareness permits people to dialogue with their thoughts and assumptions and influence them. Thus awareness grants people more freedom over those external voices that would control them.[13]

Thus, the goal of spiritual intervention is to enable awareness, to encourage it. The process of helping the patient to this awareness should not be coercive or overly aggressive. However, it is appropriate, when free information is offered, to elicit more information and then, in collaboration with the patient, to set priorities for attention. Such an approach, if it does not deflect or ignore the agenda of the patient, is proper for the clinical setting.[14] Using active listening skills, the clinician can help the patient identify their perspective of their illness. They can help uncover key stressors or issues. They can listen for themes in the patient's stories. The clinician can, by helping bring feelings to the surface, help the patient become aware of, and deal with, disempowering thinking.

People often resist the dawning of self-awareness. The thoughts and feelings people repress are frequently dark and uncomfortable. People deny them in order to avoid being overwhelmed by them. Perhaps it is the fear that these issues cannot be resolved, that the feelings are too powerful that causes people to retreat within themselves. But spiritual health depends on awareness. As people become aware of their issues and are able to own their feelings, then they can address them and contend with them and influence them. Awareness is not the only goal of spiritual intervention, but it is a first step. As one gains more self-knowledge, then that knowledge can be evaluated, and hopefully this evaluation will result in change and growth.

From a theological perspective, awareness is not merely the process of self-dialogue, but also the process of exploring who we are in the context of the divine or sacred. The great American theologian Reinhold Niebuhr explores this concept in his book *The Self and the Dramas of History*. Niebuhr focuses on humanity as created in the image of God, *imago Dei*. For Niebuhr, the person who is truly aware is the one who recognizes the *imago Dei* in his or her life.[15] If we expand this concept to include an awareness of the divine or sacred in each person, this is a concept that has wide acceptance. Awareness then is to see oneself from a transcendent perspective, to see the self in the context of something larger and more powerful. To see one's self in the context of that which gives not only the individual life, but all of life meaning. Sometimes it is this transcendent perspective that allows people to get a clear picture of themselves. It is this perspective that allows people to contradict their negative self-perceptions and grasp their potential.

Questions for reflection

- Can you remember a moment when, for some reason, you suddenly saw yourself in a new way?
- How did this new insight occur? In what way was a 'mirror' placed in front of you?
- When you look in the mirror, what do you normally see? Someone you accept or someone you judge?
- What is the standard by which you measure yourself? Is this measure appropriate or realistic?
- How do you respond when you 'see' something you don't like in yourself?

Amplification

Asked about their objectives when working with patients, many chaplains responded by noting that they hoped to give clients something to think about.[16] This objective fits nicely between those of awareness and reframing. Awareness is the process of helping the patient become aware of existing thoughts, feeling, perceptions, and values. Reframing is helping the patient take their new awareness and think differently about their problems. When a patient reframes, they take their self-awareness and begin to make decisions about values and beliefs. They begin to make decisions about what is helpful and facilitating and what is complicating and obstructing. They begin to experience spiritual change. But somewhere in this process there is a place for adding depth and complexity to the dialogue. This requires a combination of curiosity and patience. It is more aggressive than the process of merely gathering information. With amplification, our questions seek to add depth to what is being explored. One question leads to another as the richness of the issue unfolds. Howard Clinebell, a major figure in the development of faith-based counseling, talks about what he calls 'probing.'[17] Probing is 'a response which indicates the counselor's intent is to seek further information, provoke further discussion along a certain line, to query.'

In some cases, the process of amplification may paradoxically involve narrowing the field of inquiry. Many people are vague when introducing an issue that is important to them and present the problem in very broad terms. Sometimes it is useful to break the issue down into smaller pieces, finding the critical aspect that holds the key to resolution and change.

At times, it may be helpful to expand a statement and push it to its logical conclusion. 'So if you believe this, then is that also true?' At this point the clinician is not asking the patient to move spiritually, but is creating the foundation for such change.

Again, what separates amplification from awareness is the way the clinician intentionally pushes the issue. There is still a reliance on 'free,' unforced information, but the questions are slightly more directive. Amplification is an objective focused more on content of information than on feelings.

Agnes lay on her hospital bed, face turned away from her surgeon. Through her pillow she spoke.

'I'll tell you the same thing I told that nurse. Go away. I don't want your damn medications, and I don't want to talk. I just want to be alone.'

'I'm sorry you feel that way,' responded the physician. 'Often when people have had cancer surgery they want to talk to someone.'

'I have no one,' retorted Agnes.

'Really?' answered the physician. 'I thought you had several children?!'

'Forget them,' she replied. 'As far as they are concerned I'm already dead.'

'Already dead?'

'Maybe they just wish I was dead. They certainly act like I'm dead,' said Agnes.

'In what ways?' queried the physician.

'They never visit,' she replied, 'and when they come it's almost as if they can't get through the door. They instantly want to leave. They don't say much. They just sit there and squirm, then run out the door. I've got no one, I might as well die.'

'When we first met,' the doctor said, 'we talked a little about your church, and your faith. Is there any support there?'

'No!' snapped Agnes.

'It sounds like something is troubling you there, can you tell me more?'

'God doesn't care. He's given up on me just like everyone else.'

'I'm wondering,' the physician replied, 'why you feel that way?'

'Look at me,' she replied. 'God has done nothing. I've had surgery, it didn't work, I'm going to die, my family is ignoring me, and God doesn't care.'

'It sounds like you are feeling abandoned, is that right?' [perception check]

'That's right.'

'How do you see God showing you he cares?' [query, seeking amplification]

'He didn't heal me.'

'So you believe that the only way God could show you he cares is by healing you?' [expansion]

'Well...'

The conversation continued with the physician challenging Agnes' concept that God had abandoned her. He kept challenging her by asking her to define what God's love would look like or feel like. Agnes had developed a very narrow definition of what God's presence would look like in her case. By getting her to expand this definition, he was able to create an environment in which reframing was possible, where Agnes could accept God's presence and love by finding that presence in a new way. The end result was that she was able to become more open to her caregivers and her family, who loved her, but had no idea how to relate to her terminal condition.

Amplification is an objective that should be treated with great sensitivity because it moves into the realm of content. Any time we address content, we must deal with the fact that people believe different things, and that beliefs affect people in different ways. To amplify the information offered is to understand more clearly what the beliefs and perceptions are, and how they are affecting the patient. It is also a chance to get the client to explore their thoughts more deeply. It is not the job of the clinician to judge the perception, value, or belief, but to understand it. Sometimes this kind of reflection will create the potential for reframing, and at other times the belief will simply be affirmed.

Questions for reflection

- Can you think of three instances when the revealed perceptions of a patient were such that you wanted to 'dig deeper'?
- How did you respond to that desire?
- What are the dangers of seeking amplification?
- What are the benefits?

Reframing

Encouraging self-awareness is not an end in itself. Although self-awareness is, in itself, therapeutic, it is probably best seen as the beginning of a process. If the process of self-awareness reveals positive factors, then those elements should be reinforced, encouraged, and supported. If a person becomes aware, for example, through their illness, that they are connected in a loving and powerful way to other people, then the connections can be celebrated and enhanced.

If, however, what emerges from the person is troublesome and is limiting or destructive, then reframing may be needed. Reframing is a transformation of the person's point of view – about themselves, their illness, or even their faith. The goal is not merely a matter of a 'change of mind,' a mental shift, although that may be part of it. Instead, the objective should be what Elfie Hinterkopf calls a 'felt shift.' A felt shift is often marked by physiological release or relief and emerges out of the discovery of new meanings and answers generated by self-awareness.[18] It is a matter of psychospiritual growth.

When such a shift occurs, it is often just the beginning of a process. A shift from one point of reference, a change of one specific perspective, will often lead to broader and more pervasive changes. One author refers to the broad way in which a person is changed by such a shift as a wider application or global application. He says that 'the individual is often flooded by many different associations, memories, situations and circumstances' following a moment of reframing.[19] In other words, they will take their new understanding and new perspective as it relates to one specific situation, and broaden the application of their new insight to other situations. For example, a person who comes to an understanding of a negative spiritual event in their past may also understand how that event has affected many subsequent moments both in terms of feeling and actions.

Jude was a 50-year-old male who was having trouble urinating. He frequently felt the urge to urinate but was unable to do so. He knew that he should probably discuss this problem with his doctor, but found himself unable to actually make an appointment. One day, due to an accident, he found himself in the doctor's office receiving care from a nurse practitioner. Somehow, in the process of working with this sensitive provider, he found himself sharing his rather mysterious struggle. The NP, instead of scolding him for his failure to make an appointment, continued to listen and ask questions. Eventually it emerged that at one point, many years earlier, this man had been the focus of an intervention for alcohol abuse. The intervention had taken place at a doctor's office, and had been an event of great shame for this man. Indeed, it had created a significant spiritual crisis for him, causing him to feel as if he had failed God. He had felt at the time, and this feeling had been reinforced by the subsequent loss of a job and other negative outcomes, that the intervention was a personal indictment that invalidated his life and career up to that point. Although he had eventually been told that his struggles were the result of an illness, he had never been able to let go of the feelings generated by that intervention. Through his conversation with this provider he was able to go back and reframe this event, seeing it as the first step in a process of recovery instead of a negative event that invalidated much of his life. He also began to understand how this event, being unresolved, had affected him at a spiritual level every time he visited a physician's office. Each visit re-ignited the feelings of shame he felt at that intervention, and, if he managed to make an appointment, he found himself defensive and closed. He found himself assuming that any physical problem was his fault.

The critical nature of reframing lies in the fact that many people have lost their ability to have multiple views of problems or issues. With reframing, the alternatives are explored, identified, and reintroduced as possibilities. The person is offered a 'different view of the problem.'[20] They are enabled to explore multiple views of reality. Some common themes that occur when people experience illness are presented below in the form of spectrums or complements.[21]

Table 6.1

Life		Death
Openness		Secrets
Wanting to know		Not wanting to know
Hope		Hopelessness
Past	Present	Future
Resentment of dependence		Fear of abandonment
Separateness		Involvement
Relationships with family of origin		Relationship with family of affiliation
Individual concerns		Family concerns
Change		Preservation

Reframing is exploring the problem in the context of the complement. If a person is overwhelmingly focused on death, reframing seeks to introduce the complement of life. If a person is frozen, and totally committed to preservation, reframing explores change. We have already explored the concepts of spiritual spectrums (*see* Chapter 4). Reframing is ensuring that people can envision both ends of these spectrums, as well as the more general ones listed above. This allows the patient to discuss the complementary aspects; to explore, for example, both the idea that they are cursed and the idea that blessing is still possible in the midst of difficult, even tragic, times.

In most cases reframing will focus on the content of a person's thoughts or perceptions. Does a person perceive an event as hopeless or hopeful, are they feeling connected or disconnected? In some instances, however, the focus may be on context rather than content. In those moments the question is not 'What feelings are possible, and what do those feelings mean in this context?' but rather 'In what context might his feeling or perception be positive, constructive?' A person who is feeling disconnected, for example, may experience a very negative state if the context is alienation from people who are valued or helpful. But such a sense of disconnection may be not only appropriate, but actually therapeutic in the context of a controlling and minimizing relationship.

Most theories from the world of psychotherapy consider a change of perspective to be the key element in the process of healing. In the dynamic theory of therapy (Freud and Jung), awareness leads people to adapt a new perspective, a shift which then generates change. In the dynamic theory people who are in a state of dis-ease have overemphasized one side of the spectrum and ignored, perhaps totally denied, the other. Healing begins to happen when the people begin to become aware, get back in touch with this denied side. The desired outcome of reframing is a more comprehensive self.

With the social learning theory of therapy (Skinner), the focus is on how the environment or context rewards, or fails to reward, behavior. To create change, one alters the environment to create a system of rewards that lead to behavioral transformation. This still involves reframing, as the patient is challenged to look at the complement as an alternative. This kind of approach is well illustrated by the saying common in alcohol and drug recovery programs, 'If you keep doing what you are doing, you will keep getting what you are getting.' Reframing suggests an exploration of alternative contexts, and thus alternative behaviors. If a specific environment encourages drug use, the club scene for example, which then leads to drug use and to negative consequences, an alternative environment might be sought. That alternative might be a supportive family, which discourages drug use, an environment that leads to abstinence and thus to subsequent positive behaviors and consequences.

The existentialists and phenomenological therapists such as Carl Rogers insist that it is critical for patients to have radical awareness. They must not deny any experiences or perceptions. The patient's feelings about those events are critical. The goal of the therapist is to help the patient reframe (or label) those feelings in such a way as to create meaning. Anger, for example, is reframed and is no longer simply seen as 'bad.' It is instead reframed and understood as a sign that the person has a powerful need for respect. It is this change of meaning that opens the possibility for growth and development. But again, as in the other theories, a shift or reframe is the key to movement.

Cognitive therapy also believes that changes in perspective are a key component in the therapeutic process. By reframing, shifting a person's core assumptions, one changes the way that person sees reality. If a person is in spiritual or emotional dis-ease, it is often these core assumptions that contribute to the distress. Reframing the assumptions, rules, or underlying beliefs changes the way the world is viewed and can lead to relief. The goal is to replace inflexible or negative assumptions with ones that are flexible and enabling.[22]

Questions for reflection

Look back at the emotional spectrums presented in this chapter, or at the spiritual spectrums listed in Chapter 4. Choose three spectrums or complements where you have a lack of balance.

- How does being out of balance limit you?
- Think about the opposite end of that spectrum. What would it look like if you were to move toward that end of the spectrum?
- How would it feel if you made that shift?

Creation of options

As has been reflected in all of these theories of counseling, self-awareness and reframing should lead naturally to change. Awareness and reframing should cause resolution, spiritual movement, and ultimately healing. Although it is not the role of the clinician to provide the answers for the patient, helping to create awareness and challenging the client to reframe are a catalyst for change. And once the process has begun, it is appropriate to work with patients to define options for the future, and then, once the alternatives are identified, to support them in the process of choosing and implementing an option.

The healthcare context is one in which many people feel very powerless. The equipment, the terminology, the entire environment is alien, and often frightening. Decisions are frequently made for the patient who does not have the knowledge to understand or the emotional strength to resist. In addition, the disease that afflicts people can actually rob them of options, taking away autonomy. By working with patients to help them create choices in this marginalizing environment, we enhance their sense of empowerment. Sometimes, the only choices lie in the realms of the spiritual, emotional, or relational. A person who has a condition that is not responding to treatment may not have many choices about what happens in the physical realm. But they have many choices about how they will cope, about how they will choose to relate to those close to them, and about how they will invest their illness, even their death, with meaning.

Carl was a 48-year-old male who was suffering from lymphoma. He had received aggressive treatment, but it was clear that his disease was not responding and that he was nearing death. During his hospital rounds, Carl's family physician talked with him. The physician asked him if he understood what was happening. Carl responded by saying, 'Yes, nothing has worked and I know I'm going to die soon.'

The physician, using the BATHE format (*see* Chapter 7), asked him how he was feeling about the news.

'It's pretty grim,' replied Carl, 'but I think I'm doing OK. I'm pretty tired of living this way, and death doesn't seem too bad at this point.'

A few more moments of conversation revealed that Carl was a man with a strong faith, and had a very empowering view of death as a transition. The physician then asked a very creative question. 'What is the most difficult thing about your situation?'

Carl responded quickly. 'Being in this hospital! I'd really like to go home, and be able to look at my garden and have my cats around.'

The physician worked with the specialist treating Carl to enable him to return home. They negotiated an appropriate plan and Carl returned to his garden, his cats, and a supportive circle of friends who visited him, read to him, prayed with him, and even sang for him. Carl died in a warm and embracing environment, spiritually nurtured and coping well.

The task of creating options is a skill that necessitates some specific attitudes and behaviors. A major barrier to this process is impatience. The objective is to address the most significant issues, and to do so in a manner that leaves the control of the process with the patient. Impatience often causes clinicians to grab hold of the first issues that emerge. These initial issues are not unauthentic, but they may not be the most important. They are the surface issues, those it is safe to share while the therapeutic relationship is being established. The root issues will emerge more quickly in a long-term continuity relationship built over time, in which trust has already been established. Impatience can also cause the clinician to convey the meaning, albeit indirectly, that it is not 'good' or 'appropriate' for the patient to have the feelings or issues that concern him. With patience, the physician is able to illustrate that problems are a natural part of life, and that coping with those problems is also normal. Patience also keeps the healer from being too dominant in the process. It allows for a more authentic collaborative process.

The process of creating options has a number of phases. The first involves gathering information, and assessing it. It is important that both aspects of this first phase be present. It is critical to gather enough information, to not circumvent that process. It is also important to think about the information gathered rather than rushing precipitously into problem solving. The problem or issue must be defined. The third step is to work creatively with the patient to identify what positive alternatives are present, and explore them thoroughly. It is rarely wise to decide on one alternative until the full range of possibilities has been explored. Failing to create multiple options increases the chance that a poor choice will be made. Often the first choice is strongly influenced by the very emotions and issues that are impacting the patient. Looking for choices creates an opportunity for the patient to create emotional and spiritual distance from the problem. As part of this process it is also important to address the issue of responsibility or accountability. Whose problem is it really? Is it an issue that belongs to the patient, or does the responsibility really lie with someone else? Who can actually address the issue?

Anne was very upset. Several days earlier she had been involved in a car accident that had taken the life of her sister. She had been driving through an intersection when her small car was hit by a large pickup driven by an intoxicated young woman. The woman had been involved in an alcohol-enabled fight with her boyfriend and had left their apartment, about two miles away, in a rage. Anne was struggling with tremendous feelings of guilt. Although she had been driving within the speed limit and both she and her sister had been wearing their restraints, her father, in anguish over his other daughter's death, had said things that she interpreted as blame. Her mother had collapsed. The family minister, who led the parent's extremely conservative Christian church, had been challenging Anne's relationship with her boyfriend, arguing that the fact of their living together was a serious sin, punishable by God. Swirling in her head was her own sense of guilt, the concept that the accident was somehow connected to sinful behavior, and the blaming attitude of her father. During a visit, a hospital chaplain was able to help Anne identify her options, which included accepting blame and seeing the accident as a message from God. In a very short time, however, the chaplain was able to help her accept another option. That it was a tragedy caused by the choices of another person. After accepting this option, she was able to comfort her father, and find meaning in her sister's death by getting involved in a local domestic violence program. She realized that the conflict between the woman and her boyfriend was the genesis of the event, and came to accept that the real work that needed be done was by the young woman in the pickup.

The act of creating options is rarely a one-time event. Choices about treatment become choices about recovery. Choices about the meaning of the illness become choices about how to affirm life and move forward, sometimes in the context of illness. So the objective of creating choices needs to been seen as that of helping the patient to create and make choices on an ongoing basis.

Finally the process of creating options must include some discussion of consequences. If the person makes certain choices, what are the implications or likely consequences? In some cases, the consequences are clear and direct. If a person suffers from emphysema and chooses to smoke, then the costs are pretty clear. But often it is more complicated than that. A choice to practice a health behavior that damages the body may have spiritual consequences if the person sees care of the body as a spiritual activity. It may have further consequences if it impacts other people, and affects significant relationships. If the person is a parent, what is the impact on the children? What are the spiritual and emotional implications of that impact?

Questions for reflection

Think back to a time when you were in a difficult situation.

- Did you feel you had options?
- If you did feel you had options, what process did you use to identify those options?
- How did you make your ultimate decision?
- What kind of support would have enabled you to make a choice?
- What does this teach you about how to help others create options?

Empathy and support

A major key to the integration of medicine and spirituality is the development of a trusting relationship. For people to share their deepest feelings, for them to be able to express spiritual issues, they must feel safe. This means that a major objective of integration should be to create an environment of empathy. There is a difference between sympathy and empathy. If one is sympathetic they feel *for* the other person. They hear the story and feel pity, or sorrow, or anger. With empathy we feel *with* the other person. If a person has experienced loss, it is more appropriate to say we feel their sorrow rather than to say we feel sorry for them. We might also connect with them in such a way that we can identify with the breadth of their emotion. We might feel the sorrow they experience over the death of a loved one, but also the warmth they felt and still feel for that loved one. The good empathizer must respond to the other in a manner that lets them know they were understood. This focus on the patient's feelings, rather than on his/her actions or circumstances encourages the patient to explore the core of the problem.

Another way of thinking about empathy is to suggest that the listener focus on the process of the communicative event rather than on the words. The empathic listener takes in everything: words, tone, body language, and context. In other words, the listener moves, as much as is possible, into the other person's world. They work to be 'inside looking out' rather than 'outside looking in.'

One therapist suggests that empathy is not only moving into the world of the patient, but allowing the patient to move, at least slightly, into the world of the healer. She reflects this belief by saying that a 'true healing relationship also is one in which the healer and patient "look each other in the eye".'[23] Creating an environment of empathy then is not a matter of standing back objectively, but of engaging the other and engaging in mutual sharing. Healing happens when the healer is able to hear and understand the patient, and when the patient has been able to hear and understand the healer. If the patient does not feel that he or she is authentically known by the healer, then the ability of the healer to meet the other objectives of integration, such as awareness, reframing, and the identification of options, is limited. Of course there is a limit to what the healer shares and any self-disclosure must always be given with the patient as the point of focus. No patient wants to leave a clinical session feeling that they have been talked to rather than heard, that the focus of the interaction was the thoughts and feelings of the healthcare provider instead of their own. So care must be taken and boundaries and limits respected. But still the sharing should occur, if for no other reason than to model openness and authenticity.

The empathic environment can also be clarified by exploring behaviors that prevent empathy. One such behavior is a clinician projecting his or her own agenda on the patient. A physician who tries to impose his own religious agenda on a patient in order to shape or change behavior would be destroying empathy and engaging in judgment and projection. Another version of this error is being so focused on the biomedical agenda that the patient's needs are ignored. One physician was so determined, for example, to provide information about a patient's illness that he totally missed the patient's agonizing concern over the impact of the illness on his spouse. After several attempts, the patient finally stopped trying to share this concern, but he also stopped listening to the physician. He became resistive and non-compliant. The physician, rushed and distracted, did not create an empathic environment. In the end it cost time rather than saved it, and the outcome was put at risk.

Another behavior that violates the concept of empathy is the listener telling the speaker what they [the speaker] feel or believe. Listeners can help draw forth information and facilitate understanding. They can 'reflect' what comes forth, feed back what they notice. They can make guesses, and share them tentatively. But the listener cannot ultimately know what the other thinks or feels. We cannot present our perceptions as fact. One nurse, while working with a dying patient in a hospice scenario, said to a woman ravaged by breast cancer, 'I know you feel angry.' The patient responded scathingly. 'You have no idea how I feel. It is my body not yours. It is my breasts that are gone, not yours. It is my death not yours. You are not me. You have not been through what I am going through. You have no idea how I feel.' The irony is that the nurse was, as later conversations revealed, correct. But imposing her own feelings the way she did caused the patient to feel violated.

Perhaps the most critical error that destroys empathy is simply not being truly 'present' for the patient. If physicians allow themselves to be distracted by the biomedical agenda, by the stress of a full schedule, by personal issues, or by any other factors, and do not focus on their patient's agenda, empathy is destroyed. One medical social worker was talking to a patient who was struggling with some powerful ethical issues related to a sexually transmitted disease. It had been a busy day and the clinician was running behind schedule. She made the mistake of repeatedly looking at her watch. The patient was very clear in his feedback. He used good communication skills to describe the dynamics of the interaction. 'You have looked at your watch five times in the last fifteen minutes. It feels as if your schedule is more important than me. I'm out of here.' He got up and walked out.

Some might suggest that the development of empathy is really an intervention not an objective. Perhaps it is both. Others would suggest that this particular objective ought to be listed first. There is certainly merit to this idea. Empathy is foundational. It is at the heart of the entire process. It is a prerequisite for information gathering, assessment, and intervention. However, we like to put it at the end as a key reminder that all we do must be centered on the patients, on their needs, fears, and hopes. It is no accident that empathy is the 'final word' in both the BATHE technique and in the HOPE questions (*see* Chapter 7).

Questions for reflection

- Think back to a time when you felt really heard and understood. What was it about that encounter that created that empathic environment?
- Think back to a time when you did not feel heard, but instead felt manipulated or coerced. What were the factors in that encounter which made you feel that way?
- In which encounter would you have been most likely to have disclosed spiritual struggles?

The 'anti-goals'

Just as there are objectives we wish to accomplish, so, as we address spirituality in the healthcare context, there are false objectives that are inappropriate. Probably the most obvious 'anti-goal' would be the use of the healthcare encounter for proselytizing. When spirituality is addressed in the healthcare context, the focus must always be the spirituality of the patient, not the clinician. For clinicians to project or impose their spiritual agendas or values on the patient violates professional boundaries. One reason this is so dangerous is because of the power differential between the clinician and the patient. Many people endow clinicians with a great deal of power. The knowledge gap between patients and those who are caring for them, the frightening nature of the medical environment, and the vulnerability created by disease all intensify this issue. Post, Puchalski, and Larson make this point in an article on professional boundaries:

> Furthermore, the physician's potentially religious use of 'Aesculapian power' (Asklepios was the ancient Greek god of healing) might result in coercion of patients or the perception on the patient's part of an even greater power than would occur without such religious sanction...
> Adding a sacred or religious mystique to the power of the physician is suspect.[24]

Preventing one's own spirituality from simply emerging in a therapeutic encounter can be difficult, especially if spirituality plays a powerful role in one's life. The process of respecting boundaries is made even more difficult since the pressure to ignore the boundaries may originate with the patient. Patients want physicians to address spiritual issues[25] and even perform such spiritual functions as prayer.[26] This provides an incredible temptation for those clinicians with a strong spiritual perspective to share that perspective with patients.

The second false objective that should be avoided is that of providing in-depth spiritual counseling. The proper objectives for the clinician who would integrate spirituality and medicine address only the early stages of the spiritual counseling process. The clinician appropriately looks for signs of distress, helps the patient become aware of their dis-ease, helps them understand the nature of that disease, and provides empathy and support. In essence, the clinician becomes a catalyst for change. In some cases this may be enough. Once the patient has gotten in touch with their spiritual stress, they can sometimes move forward on their own, and in some cases effect their own healing.[27] But in other instances this is not the case. The problems may be too complex or too profound for the patients to move forward on their own. In these instances, the appropriate objective is for the patient to be connected with another resource with greater expertise. For a physician, who is not trained in spiritual matters (as is a pastor, rabbi, or other spiritual professional), to attempt to offer formal spiritual counseling is no more appropriate than moving beyond his or her range of expertise in the biomedical sphere. When a patient appears to need ongoing spiritual expertise, then the most appropriate response is referral, with patient consent, to an appropriate spiritual professional. We will explore this intervention in more depth in a later chapter.

Summary

The old adage is certainly true, 'if you aim for nothing you will hit it every time.' We have affirmed that the overall goal of addressing spirituality in the healthcare setting is to bring spiritual growth and healing to the patient as part of a holistic process of healing. We have identified a set of objectives which, if met, will help meet this goal. The principal objectives of spiritual integration are self-awareness, amplification, reframing, the creation of options, and empathy. These objectives should be attained using a sensitive and patient-centered approach. A final question remains. What strategies or interventions can be used to meet these objectives? Over the next three chapters we will explore the major steps which, if we use them properly, can help us accomplish those objectives. Those steps include gathering information, making a spiritual assessment, and offering a spiritual intervention.

Notes

1 Nouwen H (1997) *Seeds of Hope*. Durback R (ed.) Image Books/Doubleday, New York, NY, pp.98–9.
2 Graigie F and Hobbs R III (1999) Spiritual perspectives and practices of family physicians with an expressed interest in spirituality. *Fam Med*. **31**(8): 578–85.

3   Ellis M, Vinson D and Ewigman B (1999) Addressing spiritual concerns with patients: family physicians attitudes and practices. *J Fam Pract*. **48**(2): 105–9.

4   Adapted from: Rodrigues B, Rodrigues D and Casey DL (2000) *Spiritual Needs and Chaplaincy Services: a national empirical study on chaplaincy encounters in healthcare settings*. Providence Health Systems, Medford, OR.

5   Post SG, Puchalski CM and Larson DB (2000) Physicians and patient spirituality: professional boundaries, competency, and ethics. *Annals of Internal Medicine*. **132**(7): 578–83.

6   Ellis M, Vinson D and Ewigman B (1999) Addressing spiritual concerns with patients: family physicians attitudes and practices. *J Fam Pract*. **48**(2): 105–9.

7   Campolo A (1983) *The Power Delusion*. Victor Books, Wheaton, IL, p.17.

8   Freud S (1961) The ego and the id. In: J Strachey (ed. & trans.) *The Standard Edition of the Complete Psychological Works of Sigmund Freud* (Vol. 19). Hogarth Press, London, pp.3–44.

9   Jung C (1970) The undiscovered self: present and future. In: H Read, M Fordham and G Alder (eds) *The Collected Works of Carl G. Jung* (Vol. 10, 2e) (Hall RFC (trans.)). Princeton University Press, Princeton, NJ, pp.247–306.

10 Rogers C (1961) *On Becoming a Person*. Houghton Mifflin, Boston, MA.

11 Propst LR (1988) *Psychotherapy in a Religious Framework*. Human Sciences Press, New York, NY, p.56.

12 Propst LR (1988) *Psychotherapy in a Religious Framework*. Human Sciences Press, New York, NY, p.57.

13 Propst LR (1988) *Psychotherapy in a Religious Framework*. Human Sciences Press, New York, NY, pp.58–9.

14 Bor R, Miller R, Latz M and Salt H (1998) *Counseling in Health Care Settings*. Cassell, New York, NY, Chapter 5.

15 Niebuhr R (1955) *The Self and the Dramas of History*. Charles Scribner's Sons, New York, NY, p.131.

16 Rodrigues B, Rodrigues D and Casey DL (2000) *Spiritual Needs and Chaplaincy Services: a national empirical study on chaplaincy encounters in healthcare settings*. Providence Health Systems, Medford, OR.

17 Clinebell HJ (1966) *Basic Types of Pastoral Counseling*. Abingdon, New York, NY, p.71.

18 Hinterkopf E (1998) *Integrating Spirituality in Counseling*. American Counseling Association, Alexandria, VA, p.55.

19 Gendlin ET (1964) A theory of personality change. In: P Worchel and D Byrne (eds) *Personality Change*. Wiley, New York, NY, pp.120–1.

20 Campbell D and Draper R (1985) *Applications of Systemic Family Therapy: the Milan approach*. Grune and Stratton, London, p.7.

21 Bor R, Miller R, Latz M and Salt H (1998) *Counseling in Health Care Settings*. Cassell, New York, NY, p.32.

22 For a more detailed discussion of theories of change see LR Propst (1988) *Psychotherapy in a Religious Framework*. Human Sciences Press, New York, NY, Chapter 5.

23 Propst LR (1988) *Psychotherapy in a Religious Framework*. Human Sciences Press, New York, NY, p.33.

24 Post SG, Puchalski CM and Larson DB (2000) Physicians and patient spirituality: professional boundaries, competency, and ethics. *Annals of Internal Medicine*. **132**(7): 578–83.

25 Ehman JW, Ott BB and Short TH (1999) Do patients want physicians to inquire about their spiritual or religious beliefs if they become gravely ill? *Arch Intern Med*. **159**(15): 1803–6.

26 King DE and Bushwick B (1994) Beliefs and attitudes of hospital inpatients about faith healing and power. *Journal of Family Practice*. **39**: 349–52.

27 For a discussion of the power of awareness and belief, see Benson H (1996) *Timeless Healing*. A Fireside Book (Simon and Schuster), New York, NY.

CHAPTER 7

First steps, gathering information

The more faithfully you listen to the voice within you, the better you will hear what is sounding outside. And only he who listens can speak. Is this the starting point of the road towards the union of your two dreams – to be allowed in clarity of mind to mirror life and in purity of heart to mold it?

Dag Hammarskold[1]

When people enter the healthcare context, they come as whole persons. They do not bring physical bodies and physical issues alone, they also bring the other aspects of the self. As we have noted earlier, all of these aspects are intrinsically related to one another, and whatever happens in one realm is likely to have an impact in the other realms. Although it is impossible to truly separate the various facets of the self from one another, it is helpful, for the purposes of this discussion, to artificially divide the person who enters the healthcare context into the various aspects of personhood. In this way we can highlight the multifaceted nature of personhood, explore the complexity of the individual who seeks healing, and illustrate the importance of a multifaceted approach.

A multifaceted approach

Generally the most obvious distress in a clinical visit will be the physical ailment. But entwined with that issue may be others, resulting from or contributing to the primary, physical ailment. Take, for example, a woman who enters the healthcare context because of severe arthritis, which is limiting the use of her hands and is making it impossible for her to continue her work as a musician. Obviously the therapeutic focus will be on the arthritis. But it is critical that the healer also understand what is happening in the other facets of the patient's personhood. Here is an example of what might be happening across the entire spectrum of this patient's being.

Table 7.1   A multifaceted view of a patient

Facet	Issue
Physical	Arthritis
Soul	Sense of worthlessness and valuelessness
Social	Severe lack of social support, isolation due to sense of valuelessness, inability to work as a musician
Spiritual	Feeling disconnected from God

It is easy to see how all of the facets of the self are interconnected, and how what is happening in one component has a pervasive impact on the whole person. What is more difficult is to understand how, in a 'normal' visit, to take this reality seriously and aid the patient in a meaningful way regarding the non-physical aspects of their disease.

Helping another person explore their inner self, including their spiritual realm, is a complicated task. Each person has a unique way of perceiving and interacting with the world and unique ways of understanding and expressing his or her version of reality. Richard Bandler and John Grindler remind us of this in their book *The Structure of Magic*:

> ... Every human being has a set of experiences which constitute his own personal history and are as unique to him as are his fingerprints... The models or maps that we create in the process of living are based on our individual experiences, and, since some aspects of our experiences will be unique to us as a person, some parts of our model of the world will be singular to each of us.[2]

This is such a key concept that it is worth repeating. If we forget this concept then it becomes too easy to take shortcuts in the information-gathering process, and to fall into the trap of stereotyping and assumptions. It is also important to remember that this unique way of seeing and understanding the world translates into behavior and attitudes.

> We as human beings do not operate directly in the world. Each of us creates a representation of the world in which we live – that is, we create a map or model which we use to generate our behavior. Our representation of the world determines to a large degree what our experience of the world will be, how we will perceive the world, what choices we will see available to us as we live in the world.[3]

Our fundamental uniqueness is not a negative dynamic; indeed it adds a great deal of richness to life. However, it can be a barrier to communication in general and therapeutic communication in particular. Even under the best of circumstances, our differences force us to work at the process of communicating with one another. But this basic difficulty becomes even more intense when we are functioning in an atmosphere of vulnerability. When we are out of our normal environment and in a 'strange place' such as a hospital or medical office, we feel 'at risk.' When we are dealing with realities, such as illness, that touch core issues such as mortality, functionality, and morality, we feel exposed. When we feel vulnerable, because we are addressing issues of intensity such as our spirituality, our defensive mechanisms become engaged and we find ways to protect ourselves. If we choose to express our feelings, we do so in a way that makes us less vulnerable. For many people the healthcare setting is very frightening. It involves morbidity, mortality, strangeness, and perhaps even morality all in one scenario. It is not surprising that many people, in this environment are highly protective.

Protective communication

Sometimes when people are not very clear in their communication it is easy to get frustrated. We must get past this frustration and remind ourselves that they are simply being protective. In some cases, these are people who have been savaged by life. They have been ridiculed, betrayed, and battered. They have good reason to be protective. It is our job to be patient, to take the time to build trust, and to help those we work with move to the place where they can clearly articulate what is happening in the various facets of their personhood. At the very least it is our job to begin the process.

Indirect statements

There are many kinds of protective communication, perhaps the most common being indirect expressions of feeling. It is safe to say that most of us use this kind of proactive communication frequently. The concept is simple. Instead of making a feeling statement, 'I feel ...,' a person expresses the feeling in an indirect manner. An indirect expression can be offered through many modalities, including:

- body language
- action or behavior
- 'you' statements
- tone of voice
- sarcasm, name calling, inference, accusation.

Body language is a key indicator of what a person is thinking and feeling. In exploring the concept of communication we have discovered that non-verbal signs are an excellent indicator of what is going on with people. We should trust their tone of voice or body language long before we believe their words. Think of the woman who is sitting slumped in a chair. Her shoulders are sagging, her head is down, and her eyes are averted. Entering, the physician asks her how she is doing. 'Fine,' comes the reply. Clearly this person does not seem fine. Her direct communication is expressing that all is well, but her indirect communication is providing ample clues that there may well be problems.

Actions and behaviors may also be powerful tools for communication. Again, people may express a feeling through an action that they cannot put into words. A patient who frequently misses appointments may be sending an indirect message. The problem with such messages is that they are indirect, and thus have no specificity. Are they uncomfortable with their physician or counselor? Do they feel attacked and put down when they come into the clinic? Are they ashamed of themselves, of the fact that they are overweight, or have a drug problem, or haven't controlled their glucose levels? What is the message being sent by a patient who constantly returns for care, who shows up again and again with vague complaints?

'You statements' are one of the most common modes of indirect communication. A person feels angry, or frustrated, or frightened, but instead of expressing that feeling directly, they use a 'you statement' that expresses it indirectly. 'You don't care,' can express a person's feeling of abandonment by the caregiver, a sense of not being heard, or it can express anger over violated expectations or results. Like all indirect forms of communication, 'you statements' are inherently vague. 'You are a lousy doctor' is an indirect expression of feeling that reflects frustration that the person is not feeling better, or frustration that their goals for the healing process are being ignored. But it can also express anger, because the person does not feel heard, or anger at the illness. This vagueness may cause misunderstanding and, often, relational damage. A statement such as 'You are a lousy doctor' has the potential to frustrate and alienate the person receiving the message.

Everyone will sometimes use their tone of voice rather than words to reveal their true feelings. While the words express one message, the tone of voice is saying something quite different. The person whose tone is flat, depressed, sad, or angry is sending a message. Again, the problem is that the message is indirect, and thus must be 'translated.' Since even the most direct of messages demands a translation of sorts, this complication increases the potential that a message will be missed or misunderstood.

Perhaps the most destructive form of indirect communication involves a person transferring their feeling to the other in an aggressive and generally harmful way through the use of sarcasm, name calling, inference, and accusation. Frustration, disappointment, fear, even sadness can be contained in a comment such as 'All you people care about is making money!' That statement is an accusation and also includes an inference about the caregiver's motive. It is harsh and alienating, but what the person really feels is unclear.

Indirect statements can be very frustrating for both people involved in the communication. When communication is indirect, messages are misunderstood, critical messages are missed completely, feelings are hurt, and, most importantly, the therapeutic potential of the encounter is diminished. But indirect expressions can also be very helpful. We can be fairly certain that when a person uses an indirect method to express a feeling, that feeling is powerful and important and we should pay attention.

It should be noted that sometimes those who use an indirect method to express an emotion are very much aware of what is going on inside them but have chosen not to express their feelings directly. At other times these indirect messages are expressions of feelings of which these people are unaware. The feeling is simply so strong it expresses itself. In both cases, the expression is an important clue of something happening at the social, emotional, or spiritual level that demands attention.

The power of stories

Another way people give us clues about what is going on in the various facets of their person is through story. Stories are indirect, and are a convenient way to share what we are feeling without actually naming our emotion directly. Back in the mid-1970s, an older man was hospitalized with severe gastro-intestinal pain. His physicians did not believe his condition was serious, but because of a family history of cancer decided they needed to run a series of tests.

Shortly after he was admitted, his pastor visited him. During that visit the man told three stories. The first story was set in the early 1900s and had to do with a time when he and his wife were headed back to their farm from the 'big' city. They were carrying supplies in a horse-drawn sleigh and began the trip just as snow began to fall. The light snow became a blizzard and they were soon stuck in a huge drift.

Abandoning the sleigh, they began to struggle through the snow. Just as they were about to give up hope they saw the lights of a farmhouse and were able to find refuge from the storm. The next day they returned to their sleigh to find their horses dead.

The second story related to his days working on the railroad in the 1930s. He noted that the train yards in which he had toiled were now gone, replaced by a city park, and that most of his fellow workers were now deceased.

His third story had to do with a neighbor family, who, after generations on the same farm, had recently been forced to sell the land after the death of the family patriarch. It should be noted that this man himself was a rarity, and was living in the house in which he had been born over 70 years earlier. All of these stories had a common theme, that of loss. The motivating force that caused those stories to be told in that place at that time was a fear of impending death. Many years earlier this man's father had entered the hospital with similar pains. He never left, dying of cancer within weeks. The clues were in the stories, and by listening, a powerful and healing conversation transpired. What are the stories you hear? Why did this person share this story in this time and in this place? If there is more than one story, is there a common thread or theme that ties them together?

Issue related clues

The most critical clues to notice are those that are very specific and content-oriented. These specific clues may be either direct or indirect (although they are often indirect) and may involve generalizations, distortions, or deletions, but they are all marked by clear spiritual content. Let us return for a moment to the spiritual issues spectrum we developed earlier. People who are experiencing a spiritual crisis will tend to offer clues about the turbulence within them. They will, in many ways, provide a starting point for the resolution of their dis-ease. Examples of what these clues might sound and look like can be found in Table 7.2.

Clues such as these are usually buried in the context of a complex interaction that includes a variety of issues and, in medical encounters, may occur during a physical examination. Such clues may emanate from more than one facet. A sense of being disconnected from the sacred, for example, may also involve a sense of detachment from family member, friends, or even members of the treatment team. In some cases the clues emerge from self-awareness, in other instances they may come from struggles of which the person is only dimly aware. Thus these clues rarely 'shout' at the listener but far more frequently 'whisper.' But it is the art of listening for and recognizing such clues that is at the heart of integrating spirituality and medicine. It is with such clues that the process of bringing healing to all facets of the person begins.

For most of us, spiritual healing happens most effectively in the context of relationship. Suffering from a sense of dis-ease we tend to seek emotional, relational, and spiritual healing by connecting with, sharing with, and working with others. L Rebecca Propst, a psychologist, expresses this dynamic in her book *Psychotherapy in a Religious Framework* when she writes:

> Emotional healing is craved by all persons... We search for the sources of
> healing by seeking out relationships. Some of us mentally go through

Table 7.2 The expression of spiritual themes

Issue/theme	Verbal clue	Non-verbal
Despair	Everything just seems so dark.	Head down, eyes averted
Hope	I don't know what I would do without God.	Good eye contact, vital affect
Helplessness	I don't know why I should bother taking my medication. Nothing will help.	Flat affect, listless
Empowerment	I have to admit I have a lot of concern about this treatment, but let's give it a shot!	Energized, participates actively in treatment planning
Anger	Why? It isn't fair this should happen to me.	Flushed, fists and/or jaw clenched
Release	I got way more upset than the situation warranted.	Slight smile, peaceful affect
Guilt/Curse	I should have known this would happen.	Slumped posture, eyes down
Restoration/Blessing	You know, in spite of all that has happened, I feel so incredibly lucky.	Open body language
Fear	What will happen to me?	Hands clasped tightly
Serenity	I know I'll be OK...	Calm, appropriate affect, not overly animated
Disconnected	My greatest fear is that they hold a funeral for me, and no one will attend.	Voice flat, face tense
Connected	I am not alone.	Sits straight in the chair, strong eye contact

our address book ostensively looking for someone to spend an afternoon with, play tennis with, or eat dinner with. What we really want is a healer, a relationship where we can feel acceptance, a relationship where we can get rid of the residues. For many of us, there are moments of despair when we realize that there are very few of those relationships in our lives.[4]

One of those healing relationships can be, and should be, the relationship between healthcare professionals and those they seek to serve. The clinical encounter should be a truly therapeutic encounter where a healing partnership is formed and the process of examination, discovery, and change can begin. This is, in essence, what the integration of spirituality and healthcare is all about – helping people who are suffering from disease, and potentially dis-ease, to examine themselves, discover their inner issues, express critical feelings, and move toward change and healing.

Active listening helps develop the healing partnership and facilitates change. First, it creates value in the person who is sharing their thoughts and feelings. If we are trained to listen, our agenda is to hear the other, to focus on them and their agenda, their ideas, feelings and concerns. Physicians, for example, are trained to gather information. But in general they seek to control the conversation, and the dialogue is designed to meet their needs, not the needs of the patient. All too rarely, the patient is given the free and friendly space to share that which is within. It feels incredible when it happens, and people end up feeling enabled, empowered, and valued. Listening is thus a therapeutic intervention.

Listening creates release. Our emotions are powerful and must be expressed. The more powerful the emotions, the more joyful or painful, the more difficult it is for us to put them into words. To share those powerful feelings makes us vulnerable. To put our feelings 'out there' for human consumption places us at risk. That is one reason we tend to codify our feelings in such creative ways. But the expression of such feeling is in itself cathartic. There is power in such self-disclosure.

Listening creates awareness. Many times we do not fully understand what is happening within the various aspects of the self. Without warning issues build to the point that we begin to 'act out.' Our inner issues express themselves through our words and actions. A good listener helps us 'hear' ourselves and begin to understand what is happening spiritually, emotionally, or relationally. George Herbert Mead, a major figure in American philosophy and one of the founders of Pragmatism (along with Dewey), put it this way in the book *Mind, Self and Society*: 'We see ourselves as we see other people seeing us.' One young pastor was once brought up short by a question posed by a member of his church: 'What are you angry about?' As questions go, it was not perfect, as it made an assumption about what the pastor was feeling. But the ensuing conversation was enabling and revealing. The immediate response to the question was another question, 'Why do you think I'm angry?' 'Because your last couple of sermons have felt angry! Normally your talks are very positive, but the last two or three have been almost hostile.' It was as if a mirror had been put in front of this minister. After some honest reflection he was forced to admit, he was angry, infuriated by a community struggle that was creating significant issues for his church. He had not been aware of that anger, but the message had been coming through loud and clear. It took another, helping him hear his own words, his own tone, to bring the simmering anger to awareness. That awareness was a prerequisite to resolution and healing.

Listening puts us in touch with inner resources. Sometimes, as we explore the topic of integration and think about the impact of spirituality on the healing process, we focus on the negative end of the spectrum. Despair gets more attention than hope. But listening can help the healer and the person suffering from illness to get in touch with those positive factors present within their emotional, relational, or spiritual facets. It is said that Martin Luther when challenged with adversity would often comfort himself by saying, 'I have been baptized.' For him his baptism was a symbol of his connection with God, and that connection was an incredible resource in times of trial. The goal of listening is not just to explore spiritual issues that may be a barrier to healing, but also to discover spiritual resources that are an aid to healing. For one cancer patient, his small Bible study group was a powerful tool. This group reinforced his sense of relationship with God and provided incredible social and emotional support. His physician wisely encouraged and supported his participation, even when it was physically difficult. A black woman, suffering from chronic pain and fatigue, found that prayer gave her a sense of empowerment and hope. Her physician, hearing her share this powerful reality, wrote her a new prescription: 'one prayer, three times daily.'

Listening can also provide the impetus for change. In many cases listening leads to awareness, awareness creates the possibility for reflection and examination, and this examination provides the foundation for a restructuring or changing of one's thoughts (mental health professionals would call this cognitive therapy). This brings us to the issue of outcomes. What are we trying to do through the integration of healthcare and spirituality? As we have discussed in Chapter 6 basic goals of integration has a lot to do with process. With integration we help people begin the process of moving on in life. Integration has the potential to help people develop personally, in all aspects of their being. Injury and illness have a powerful effect on most people. Diseases challenge our belief and values. Trauma shakes our being and forces us to reassess. Out of the therapeutic process can come not only physical healing, but spiritual, emotional, and relational growth as well. As people share and are heard, as understanding emerges, as patterns of behavior and thought are challenged, a foundation is established for growth and change.

If we look at the structure of a typical clinical encounter we can see how the use of active listening fits in as a diagnostic tool. It parallels the information-gathering stage of the clinical encounter. Listening plays the same essential role as asking for a current complaint, taking a medical history, and performing a physical exam. It is a way to get the information needed to make an assessment and develop a treatment plan.

Table 7.3 The multifaceted clinical encounter

Event	Facet	Gathering information	Reflection/assessment	Diagnosis/ definition
Onset of severe arthritis	Physical	Medical interview, physical exam	Review symptoms, test results, etc.	Arthritis
	Soul	Listening for clues	Clue: 'I'm totally worthless'	Sense of worthlessness and valuelessness
	Social	Creative questions	Observed lack of interaction with friends, lack of connection to provider, and low compliance with treatment plan	Severe lack of social support, isolation due to sense of valuelessness
	Spiritual	Specific use of spiritually focused questions	Comment about feeling 'alone,' abandoned by God	Feeling disconnected from God

Learning the language of healing

Before we move on to the topic of assessment, let us review the basic components of active listening. Very few healthcare workers, indeed very few people of any sort, have had training in active listening. Yet learning these skills is the same as learning the language of healing. These skills are not complex and yet it is important to understand that learning to use them is a process that can be frustrating.

In general there are four stages in the process of learning a skill. The first stage is that of *unconscious/incompetent*. At this stage a person neither knows the skill, nor knows how to do it. The second stage is *conscious/incompetent*. At this stage the learner has gained a basic knowledge of the skill, but really can't do it. The third stage is *conscious/competent*. At this point the person both knows the skill and can do it. However, it is not yet a comfortable process. Using the skill takes concentration and conscious effort. The final stage is *unconscious/competent*. This is the point where the learners not only know the skill, but have made it a normal part of how they function. They don't think about it, they just do it. In this case they have mastered the art of listening, and have greatly enhanced their ability to practice the art of healing.

Think about the process in terms of skiing. At the unconscious/incompetent stage the beginners stagger across the flats, boots flapping, skis askew, not knowing what to do and clearly not able to function. Then comes the first lesson. The first step is to learn what to do. So the instructor shows them how to make a wedge with their skis, a movement that will enable them to control their speed, stop, and eventually turn. They have heard the description, they have seen it demonstrated, but they haven't yet done it. They are at the conscious/incompetent stage. So they try it out. The lucky move on to the conscious/competent stage. They know what to do, and they can do it, but it takes concentration and effort. Only when they can put their feet into a wedge and, almost without thinking, slow down, stop, and turn (the unconscious/competent stage) are they ready to move on to the next skill.

Thus, learning to listen is a process. It takes time and energy. It takes practice. There will be moments when it seems incredibly awkward (especially at the conscious/competent stage). At some point, as people learn to incorporate the skills of active listening, they will feel as if the people they are listening to are painfully aware of the skills they are using, and feel manipulated. It may be true that some people will recognize the skills at work. But in most cases people are so happy to finally be heard that they don't care. It is important for the learner to be patient and not abandon the process too quickly. For if they persevere, eventually the time will come when it will simply be a part of who they are and how they function.

So let us look at some of the basic tools, and how they might be applied in the therapeutic encounter. The best place to begin when looking at tools that facilitate communication is to explore habits that hinder communication. There are innumerable behaviors that get in the way of effective listening, but the following list includes some of the most common.

Blocks to listening[5]

The 'How am I doing?' syndrome makes it hard to listen because you're always trying to assess how you are coming across to the person who is talking. 'Do I impress this person? Do they like me?' Some people get very competitive here. 'Who is smarter, more competent – me, or the other?' With this syndrome the 'listeners' can't let much in because they are too busy worrying about how they are doing! In the medical culture this syndrome may simply involve the need of the professional to establish their expertise, their unique ability. They are so busy playing doctor or nurse or therapist that they are not truly engaged in the dialogue. Authentic listening is hindered.

The **mind reader** doesn't pay much attention to what people say. In fact he/she often distrusts it. This person is trying to figure out what the other person is *really* thinking and feeling. While we advocate active listening, and the art of helping people tells us what they need to tell us, we do not advocate mind reading – making assumptions, imposing our perceptions about the other person upon them. Whenever we assign a feeling or an issue to another person there is a significant danger that we may be inaccurate. We may decide a person is angry when they are really frustrated, or fearful when they are really angry. The very process of active listening is designed to help us listen, allow the other person to pursue their agenda, and eventually reveal clearly that which is within.

We don't have time to listen when we are **rehearsing** what we are going to say. Our whole attention is on the preparation and crafting of your next comment. We have to *look* interested, but our mind is going a mile a minute because we have a point to make. Some people rehearse whole chains of responses. 'I'll say, then he'll say, then I'll say,' and so on. This is a real issue for healthcare providers, who must express and inform as well as gather information. At some point the temptation is there to stop listening, especially to patients with vague physical ailments, and to begin to rehearse what will be said. The focus becomes sharing the diagnosis, imparting critical educational material, and negotiating a treatment plan. Although all of these activities must eventually occur, healers must be careful that they do not cut the conversation short or cause it to stall at a shallow level because they are composing what they are going to say.

When we **filter** we listen to some things, and not to others. We pay only enough attention to see if somebody's angry, or unhappy, or if we are in emotional danger. Once assured that the communication contains none of these things, we let our mind wander. With patients with chronic or vague problems, particularly with people who have shared the same story or information before, the tendency may be to listen carelessly.

When we **prejudge** others and give them negative labels, we powerfully effect the way we interact with them. If we prejudge someone as stupid or nuts or unqualified, we don't have to pay much attention to what they say. We've already written them off. A basic rule of listening is that judgments should be made only *after* we have heard and evaluated the content of the message. With some patients it may be easy to put people in a category that discounts them as a person. 'He is a drug seeker.' 'She is a hypochondriac.' 'She will never change her behaviors.' When this happens we no longer treat the other with appropriate respect, and our listening becomes ineffective.

Sometimes we like to play the role of **adviser**. There is something satisfying in being the great problem-solver, ready with help and suggestions. We don't have to hear more than a few sentences before we begin searching for the right advice. However, while we are cooking up suggestions and persuading some to 'just try it,' we may miss what's most important. We didn't hear the feelings, and didn't acknowledge the person's pain. He or she still feels basically alone because we couldn't listen and just *be* there. This block is a tremendous issue for healthcare professionals, whose very role is to 'solve the problem.' All too often we stop listening too soon. We grab on to a basic complaint or issue, and never take the time to ascertain whether this is truly the main issue. To make this error is much like throwing pharmaceuticals at high blood pressure without ever looking at factors contributing to that problem, such as obesity or alcohol use. The therapeutic encounter is a process. We must be careful not to cut the process short.

When we **spar** we find ourselves arguing and debating with people. The other person never feels heard because we're so quick to disagree. In fact, a lot of our focus is on finding things with which to disagree. We take strong stands, are very clear about our beliefs and preferences. In effect we 'put down' the other person. In medical encounters physicians sometimes discount the beliefs of their patients, or discount the meaning the patients attach to their illness. If a patient says, 'I think I have cancer,' the professional may quickly discount this perspective. The intent is usually to reassure and encourage, but such an abrupt discounting of the person's beliefs says, indirectly, 'You are ignorant.' A much better response might be to ask a question, such as 'What makes you think you might have cancer?' This kind of a question may lead to a very different kind of interaction!

When we **derail** a conversation we make comments that block further conversation on that topic. We may change the subject, or laugh it off. There is a particular version of this block that is prevalent within clinical encounters. Derailing in the healthcare context often takes the form of the healthcare professional derailing the patient's agenda and replacing it with a 'medical' agenda. Instead of listening to the patient's fears, or anger, or frustration, the physician, nurse, or other professional retreats into the world of medical details, diagnosis, and treatment plans. While it is critical to inform patients about their disease, provide them with a diagnosis, and develop a treatment plan, we must be careful not to ignore deeply felt concerns or issues disclosed by the patients, either overtly or subtly.

Often, when faced with difficult people or difficult situation we **placate.** 'Right... Right... Absolutely... I know... Of course you are... Incredible... Yes... Really?' Most of us enjoy being liked. Most of us don't like confrontation. It some cases this causes us to simply agree with everything. We may half-listen, just enough to get the drift, but we are not really involved. We are placating rather than tuning in and examining what's being said. This is particularly easy to do with patients who move into realms of relationships, spirituality, and emotions. After all, this is not the main focus of the healthcare visit, so why spend too much energy on those issues? It is easier to offer pseudo compassion.

Each of us has our favorite ways of blocking communication. We can block for many reasons, and use various techniques, but normally we will find we have a pattern. Think for a moment about your standard blocking activities. List the blocks that seem typical of the ways you avoid listening.[6] You may use the list above as a guide, but be aware that the list is not all-inclusive. Appendix A contains a brief tool that may help you understand your personal 'blocking patterns.'

Questions for reflection

- What is your most commonly used block?
- With whom do you use blocking the most?
- What subjects or situations usually trigger the block?

It is important that we understand our patterns of blocking. If we do not clearly identify our blocks we will be likely to use them. Such patterns become automatic and unconscious very quickly. Our goal is not only to work systematically to create good listening habits, but to work at eliminating bad habits that have developed.

Basic listening skills

We can listen much faster than people can talk. In all of the instances above, we use the spare time that is available in our mind as we listen to engage in activities and responses that block and minimize our effectiveness. Instead of allowing this to happen, our goal should be to use time creatively, to bring our mind's capacity to bear on the words of the other, and help them say what they want and need to say – whether they know what that is or not! The authors of *Messages* say it well:

> Listening doesn't mean sitting still with your mouth shut. A corpse can do that. Listening is an active process that requires your participation. To fully understand the meaning of a communication, you usually have to ask questions and give feedback. Then, in the give and take that follows, you get a fuller appreciation of what's being said. You have gone beyond passively absorbing, you are a collaborator in the communication process.[7]

Listening is the active use of specific skills. It is a commitment to understanding and acknowledging how other people feel. It is exploring all facets of their personhood. It is working with them to define how they see the world. It is getting our own selves out of the way, at least for a moment. It is putting aside our prejudices, assumptions, values, and, especially, our agendas. Following are some key skills that can be used in the process of gathering information, and at other stages in the process of helping people address spiritual issues. These tools will be explained here in some detail. An active listening workbook that can be used by individuals or groups can be found in Appendix A.

Paraphrase is the skill of responding to the content and meaning of another person's verbal communication. It identifies with the *words* by clarifying the content for accuracy. A paraphrase can be very important in certain, specific circumstances. It is a skill that focuses on 'content' and is very useful when the speaker has shared a lot of information without allowing for a response. The paraphrase allows the listener to summarize the information and also check for accuracy. If the news is surprising or confusing the paraphrase can be used to create clarity. Sometimes, if the information demands thought, the paraphrase can provide the listener with time, or space. Finally, a paraphrase is very useful if the 'trust' factor between the two parties is low. By paraphrasing, the listener says, 'What you have said is valuable and I have really listened.' The following is an example of how a paraphrase might be used in a clinical encounter:

> **Patient:** Doctor, I am really concerned about this operation. I don't know you, and I'm not really clear about what is involved in this surgery. It seems as if there is a lot of risk and not a lot of benefits.
>
> **Physician:** I hear you saying that you are not sure about going forward with this operation. You are not clear about the details of the operation, and are not sure if the benefits justify the risk. The fact that you don't know me well also makes the decision difficult. Does that summarize your concerns accurately?
>
> **Patient:** Yes, I really am concerned and feel like I need to talk more about this. Is that OK?
>
> **Physician:** Of course it is ... [a discussion of the procedure, the risk and benefits, etc., follows]

Remember, a paraphrase should accurately restate the content of the original statement, although it is not a matter of just parroting the words. It should not infer too much, nor should it try to address the feelings behind the statement. The value of the tool is that it helps bring focus to the words of the other person and is an effective remedy to most listening blocks.

To practice this skill find a friend who is willing to do something a bit strange. Ask them to start telling you something about their day, or week. As the story unfolds respond with nothing but paraphrases. Your partner gets to tell you whether you've truly heard what they have said. Allow them to point out misunderstandings, mistakes, or assumptions. Try to use a paraphrase in a majority of your conversations, professional and personal. At first it will feel awkward and weird, but eventually you will become comfortable with its use. You will also learn to respect how this simple tool can help you hear more effectively and to demonstrate that you are listening.

In a **perception check** the listener describes what he/she perceives to be the other person's feelings to check for understanding. The goal is to translate the other person's non-verbal communication (gestures, expressions, tone of voice) into a tentative description of feelings. It is critical to understand that a perception check is tentative. We do not know what the other person is thinking or feeling, we can only guess. When we make a perception check we are sharing our guess with the other person and allowing them to affirm, deny, or adjust our perception. A good perception check conveys this message: 'I want to understand your feelings, is this [feeling word] the way you feel?' The perception check has four stages.

1 **Look and listen:** You listen to the content and look at the non-verbal clues. If there is a clash between the content of the words and the non-verbal behavior, put your trust in the non-verbal message.
2 **Think:** You try to identify a feeling. The best way to do this is to get in touch with the feelings the statement stirs inside you.
3 **Share your perception:** Make a tentative statement of what you believe the other person is experiencing.
4 **Check:** Ask a question to discover whether your guess was correct. It is not necessary that you always be right. It does help if your guess is close!

Following is an example of how a perception check might be used in a clinical encounter.

> **Patient:** You think I need surgery? I can't need surgery! (Voice rising, eyes wide, body tense)
>
> **Physician:** I sense that the idea of surgery really concerns (feeling word) you. (Perception)
> Is that right? (Check)
>
> **Patient:** Concerned! You have no idea, I'm terrified (adjustment). My dad went into the hospital when I was a child and never came out alive!

In this conversation the physician listened to the content of the patient's words and paid attention to the tone of voice and body language. If this had not occurred the physician might have responded by saying something like, 'Yes, you do need surgery, it's necessary.' This would have been a blocking statement as it would have ignored the underlying message of the patient and created a potentially adversarial position. By picking up the information offered by the patient, responding appropriately, and then allowing the patient to offer more information, the physician was able to move toward an issue which was strongly affecting the patient, a fear of surgery rooted in her childhood. As the conversation progresses, the depth of the conversation deepened further still, and the woman was able to share a powerful fear of death. The physician was able to refer her to a chaplain who was able to help her address this existential and spiritual issue.

Since a perception check is a way of validating a tentative perception, rather than the pronouncement of a fact, it is important that the statement include a 'stem' that illustrates the provisional nature of the assessment. Some of the stems that can be used are as follows:

- I get the impression that ...
- I'm wondering if ...
- It seems to me that ...
- It sounds to me as if ...
- I have a hunch that ...
- It appears to me that ...
- Is it possible that you might be feeling ...

Many people, when first exposed to the concept of a perception check, ask if the method is very contrived, and believe that those they use it with will feel manipulated. In reality, people like being heard, and appreciate the respect that is shown by a person who is willing to share his/her perceptions, and allow those perceptions to be corrected or adjusted. It must also be remembered that a perception check is rarely used in isolation from other listening tools.

> **Patient:** I am having a terrible time in my relationship with my roommate. We always seem to be getting on each other's nerves.
>
> **Physician:** So your roommate and you are having some real problems getting along? (paraphrase) I sense that this really has you frustrated (perception) ... Is that right? (check)

The goal of a perception check is simple: to move the conversation to a deeper level by giving the speaker permission to tell you how they really feel. It is not critical that you be absolutely correct, but it is nice if you are on the same end of the emotional spectrum. Once the feeling has been expressed directly, the conversation will usually move deeper as the listener can take that information and ask questions that bring deeper disclosure and understanding. An exercise can be found in Appendix A to help you practice this skill.

Behavior description is reporting specific, observable actions of other people *without* making accusations, inferences, or name calling. It is like putting a verbal mirror in front of the other person and exposing them to their tone of voice, body language, or behavior. It is a skill that can provide a foundation for deepening the discussion through the use of such skills as perception checks about behaviors, tone of voice, and body language that are major clues to what is happening at the feeling level.

It is a mistake to ignore these powerful clues. At times we may use such clues to create assumptions about what we perceive is going on, but we don't use them as a tool for helping the other tell us their story. The greatest error we make is to react to what we experience and move into inference and, in difficult situations, to accusation and name calling. Following are some examples of how behavior or body language can move us into territory that is neither enabling nor constructive.

- Fran has missed her last three appointments!
  Accusation: Fran is irresponsible.
  Inference: Fran was avoiding talking about her issues.
- The person constantly rubs her hands.
  Accusation: She is weird.
  Inference: She is nervous.
- The person averts his eyes when answering questions.
  Inference: He is being evasive.
  Accusation: He is lying.

The problem is that we really don't know why a person is behaving in a manner that is troubling. Nor do we really know what their tone or body language portrays. Again, we can only guess. To make an inference or internal accusation is to fail to respect the interpersonal gap and the complexity of the human being. To make an inference or accusation, especially if it is done publicly and not merely internally, is also a blocking action. People get defensive when they are accused of something, and they become self-protective when they believe others are trying to impose feelings or motives on them.

If we can reflect a behavior or other non-verbal clue back to the other person, it can help move the conversation forward, and deeper. Following is an example of how a behavior description can be used in a therapeutic encounter.

> **Patient:** (Sits slumped, with head down and eyes averted. Voice is flat and without energy.) Things have been OK. I've really been fine.
> **Physician:** You know, I can't help but notice that you're slumped, and you aren't looking me in the eye the way you normally do (behavior description). I am wondering if you might be feeling a bit frustrated with the problems you have been having with your diabetes. Would that be possible?
> **Patient:** Yeah, now that you mention it, I guess I have been feeling a bit down.
> **Physician:** What exactly is it that is troubling you the most ...

A behavior description can be a very powerful tool for helping people get in touch with their feelings. It can also be used to deal with people who are difficult. Sometimes by combining a behavior description with other skills we can create positive movement.

> **Physician:** Mary, I have noticed that you have missed several appointments lately. It is also clear from your blood tests that you are having trouble controlling your blood sugar (behavior description). I want you to know that I am frustrated by the fact you have missed your appointments (direct expression of feeling) because I am very concerned about your health. I am also concerned about your glucose levels. Can you tell me why you think your levels are so high? (creative question)
> **Mary:** Dr Anderson, I am so sorry I have missed my appointments. I knew my levels were high and I was embarrassed...

This conversation could have been very different if the physician had used an accusatory tone, or had projected feelings upon this patient.

> **Physician:** Mary, you have missed several appointments lately. That is very irresponsible. We are very busy here and it is unfair of you to take an appointment and not show. That means someone else can't be seen. And, as you probably know, your blood sugar is high. You clearly haven't been following your diet.

The patient in the scenario could easily get defensive, and the opportunity to work together in a therapeutic relationship would be lost. Sometimes it is difficult to separate authentic behavior descriptions from inferences, accusations, or name calling. An exercise found in Appendix A can be used to reinforce the difference between these various responses.

Creative questions are simply questions. Since our major purpose is to take the free information we are offered, and use that as a foundation for gathering more information in a non-coercive manner, creative, enabling questions are critical. However, not all questions are creative. A question is **not** creative if:

- it changes the subject
- it moves too quickly and invades private space
- it is a put-down
- it is 'loaded'
- it can be answered too easily with a 'yes' or 'no.'

It is a creative question if:

- it is congruent and flows naturally from the context of the conversation
- it prompts the other person's story
- it gives the other person permission to say more
- it uses 'free' information given and does not assume knowledge.

In general, creative questions are what are called 'open' questions. They cannot be answered with a 'Yes' or 'No' but prompt a release of more information. See Appendix A for an exercise that will allow you to practice asking creative questions.

Negative inquiry is the act of coaching the other person in their negativity. In many instances people begin criticisms and complaints at a very vague level. Often the more powerful the feeling, the more generalized or vague the comment. 'I feel "off."' 'You are a lousy doctor.' The problem is that these critical or negative statements, being too vague, don't really say anything. They are not specific enough to help us understand what the other person is struggling with, doesn't like, or desires to change. Such statements certainly don't give us enough information to decide whether the statement is valid and helpful or not. Nor do they provide information to facilitate further conversation. The goal should be to help those who are critical or negative become more specific so we can learn from them, evaluate the statement appropriately, and get to the true issue.

If the person has made a negative comment about us or a treatment plan, we must coach the person, encourage them to provide more specific criticism.

> **Physician:** I hear you saying that you don't think I'm a good doctor. What exactly is it that you don't like?

If the person cannot or will not get specific, then we need to be persistent in our attempt to get them to be more helpful.

> **Physician:** I hear your criticism, but I cannot really respond unless you are more specific. Please tell me exactly what it is about my practice of medicine you do not like.

Sometimes we will encounter a continued refusal to be more specific. In such cases it is often important to be persistent, to keep asking the speaker to get more specific. There is a limit to how aggressive we should be, and we should be careful not to be too assertive. But some persistence is appropriate.

In the same way that we should coach others in their criticisms, so we should coach them in terms of other negative comments. The drive for specificity is natural to the healing professions. If a person has an injury or illness, we do not hesitate to ask them to quantify their pain or discomfort. 'If,' we ask, 'pain is on a scale of 1 to 10, where would you place it?' This is essentially the same principle.

> **Physician:** I heard you say that you are feeling off. It would be very helpful to me if you could be more specific. If you were to use one word, besides 'off,' to describe how you feel, what would it be?
> **Patient:** I guess the word I would have to use is 'empty.'
> **Physician:** How strong is this feeling? If you were to put it on a scale from 1 to 10, where would it be?

Since, in many cases, discussion in healthcare encounters focuses on disease, this kind of negative inquiry, which is based on the skill of creative questioning, can be extremely important and transformational.

Questions for reflection

- Think about your normal pattern of relating to patients. Do you use active listening skills?
- With which of these skills do you feel most comfortable?
- Which of these skills is the most difficult for you?

Specific tools for spiritual inquiry

To this point we have been focusing primarily on free information that comes voluntarily and unsolicited from those engaged in the therapeutic process. The basic listening skills we have explored are extremely useful for identifying the clues and enable another person to disclose what is happening internally, the issues in the spiritual, social, or emotional level that are affecting their lives. Certainly one of the major times when it is appropriate for a clinical encounter to move into the spiritual realm is when a clue is presented that indicates there is a spiritual issue. However, there are several other instances when such a movement is appropriate.

One such moment is when information is being gathered as part of obtaining a personal and medical history. When a physician and patient are getting to know each other, when the therapeutic relationship is being developed, a lot of information is exchanged. Much of that information is very intimate and personal: eating habits, sleeping habits, job information, relational information, sexual activity. The goal is to get to know the whole person, to understand all the factors that may be contributing to the disease or dis-ease. If we take seriously the concept that a person is multifaceted and is spiritual, emotional, and social as well as physical, then it is appropriate to include questions in this information-gathering process that focus on the spiritual.

There are a number of mnemonics that provide appropriate and sensitive questions for exploring a person's spiritual framework. Christina Puchalski, assistant professor of medicine at George Washington University and director of the George Washington Institute for Spirituality and Health, has developed the FICA questions that can be used to explore a person's basic spiritual and religious framework.[8] Those questions are:

- Faith: What is your faith tradition?
- Important: How important is your faith to you?
- Church: What is your church or community of faith?
- Apply: How do your spiritual beliefs apply to health? How might we address your spiritual needs?

Gowri Anandarajah and Ellen Hight, assistant professors in the Department of Family Medicine at Brown University, suggest that an initial spiritual exploration should cover four areas that can be remembered with the letters HOPE.[9] Below is a description of each of these areas and a couple of sample questions for each category.

- Hope: Sources of hope, comfort, meaning, love, and connection.
  What are your sources of hope, meaning, or comfort?
  What do you hold on to in difficult times?
- Organized religion: Are you part of a religious or spiritual community? Does it help you? How?
- Personal spirituality and practices: Do you have any personal spiritual beliefs that are independent of organized religion?
  Do you have any personal spiritual practices that are important and helpful to you?
- Effects: Has being ill affected your ability to do things that help you spiritually (or has it affected your spirituality)?
  Is there anything I can do to help you access the resources that normally help you?

Several other options are available, but these are two outstanding examples of the kinds of questions that can be used during the relationship-building and information-gathering process. Some criticize this tactic, believing that such questions create a certain degree of pressure and may make people who do not consider themselves spiritual or religious uncomfortable. However, such questions 'normalize' spirituality. By including these very personal questions along with many other more traditional but just as personal questions, we let people know that they can include their spiritual self in the healing process and in their discussions with us.

There are several other times when it is appropriate for the therapeutic partnership to move over into the spiritual realm. One is when a person receives bad news. This might include news of a loss, of a terminal illness, or even news of a life-changing or chronic disease. At such a time, issues about life, death, and meaning come to the forefront. Spiritual issues emerge and need to be addressed. One group, adapting a brief intervention for smoking cessation, created an effective tool for addressing spiritual issues with patients who have been given difficult news.[10] This tool begins with a basic opening statement, and then provides a variety of options, depending on the initial response of the patient. The opening questions are as follows.

- Religious or spiritual issues often influence how patients deal or cope with... Some people find their spiritual beliefs to be very helpful, while others do not find them helpful or never really think about these things at all. I would be interested to understand how you feel about this?
- What part, if any, do your spiritual beliefs play in how you have been dealing with [define disease]?

Once these questions have been asked, the interview moves in different directions, depending upon the response of the patient. Basically the physician explores the patient's beliefs, asking questions that are appropriate for one of four basic groups. Those groups are those who:

- indicate a supportive/positive god
- have a positive but non-specific view of the sacred
- reveal spiritual conflict including anger or guilt
- reject spiritual/religious beliefs.

If, for example, the patient has a supportive and positive view of God, the physician might ask about their community of faith, specific ways in which their faith supports them, or spiritual practices. The goal would be to find ways to access faith as a healing resource. If they reveal spiritual conflict, the questions will focus on clarification of the issue, and seek to move the patient toward resolution. If the person rejects spiritual or religious beliefs the physician may well simply drop the topic as a source of conversation.

Once the inquiry about beliefs has been completed, some additional questions can be asked.

- Are there ways in which you have/can find a sense of meaning and peace through all of this?
- Is there anyone else you can talk to?

The final step in the 'intervention' is to explore the availability of other resources. In other words, who can the patient turn to? A friend? A spiritual leader? Guides for physicians are available that provide healthcare professionals with an outline of this exploratory process.[11]

Another time when it is logical to move into the realm of the spiritual is when a chronic or long-term problem is entering its final stages in which complications begin to occur, such as depression, chronic pain, diabetes, arthritis, or neurological syndromes. These are very difficult conditions that wear at the fabric of a person's being and often create spiritual distress. In such instances the BATHE tool may be very effective.[12] This technique was designed for use in the modern clinical environment and is intended to fit within a 15-minute appointment. The framework is relatively simple, but allows for many possible variations. The basic structure of the interview is as follows.

- **Background:** What is going on in your life? (the context of the visit)
- **Affect:** How do you feel about what is going on? What is your mood? (allows the patient to label current feeling state)
- **Trouble:** What troubles you the most? (helps focus and bring out the symbolic significance of the event/illness)
- **Handling:** How are you handling that? (assessment of functioning)
- **Empathy:** This must be very difficult. (builds trust and the therapeutic relationship)

The first area of inquiry focuses on the life situation of the patient. This technique assumes, for the most part, an ongoing relationship between the healthcare professional and the patient. Normally the professional will ask a simple, leading question such as, 'What has happened since your last visit?' In this question the healer expresses many things, including interest and compassion. The second question is extremely important. It allows the person with the disease to share how the illness, injury, or chronic condition is affecting them. It is an opportunity to move the discussion to the level of feeling. If the relationship between the provider and patient is long-standing, and one of trust, the patient may be fairly direct. In many cases, however, the answer will be indirect and the healer will need to use active listening skills to get to the core feeling.

The third question, 'What troubles you the most?', endows the patient with a degree of power. It allows them to set the agenda for the conversation and for the treatment plan itself. This question allows the person to define their goal for therapy. That goal may or may not be the one assumed by the healthcare professional. The nurse may want to focus on pain, the patient on functionality. The physician may believe that the terminal nature of a condition is the issue, while the patient may be more concerned about the impact of his disease on his family.

The focus then turns to how the patient is handling the situation. This question shows respect for the patient and his or her coping mechanisms. It not only allows the physician, nurse, or therapist to ascertain whether the patient is coping, but also to support those coping strategies that are working. In other words, by exploring current coping, the opportunity is created to either support effective coping strategies or introduce new strategies, or both.

The final movement in the interview is one of empathy. It is important for the healthcare professional to let their patients know that they have been heard, that they are understood and supported, and that there is true compassion.

Summary

Movement into the realm of the spiritual can take place at several logical moments in the healing process. It can happen when the patient and physician begin the process of gathering and sharing information. It can happen at a moment of crisis or loss. It can occur regularly, as a normal part of a long-term process, or when the patient offers specific clues.

The movement can involve the use of tools designed specifically for this purpose, such as the FICA questions or the HOPE questions. It might involve the use of more general skills, such as active listening. Or it might involve a therapeutic technique such as BATHE.

In all cases the movement begins with an exploration of the spiritual aspect of the person. It is primarily a matter of gathering information, just as information is gathered about a physical issue. Once the information is gathered, then it must be analyzed, and from that analysis a plan should evolve. It is to the process of analysis that we now must turn. We have heard the stories – identified the feelings. But what does it all mean? How do we think about this information? Where do we go from here?

Notes

1   Hammarskjold D, Sjoberg L and Auden WH (trans.) (1964) *Markings*. Alfred A Knopf, New York, NY, p.13.

2   Bandler R and Grinder J (1975) *The Structure of Magic*. Science and Behavior Books, Palo Alto, CA, p.12.

3   Bandler R and Grinder J (1975) *The Structure of Magic*. Science and Behavior Books, Palo Alto, CA, p.7.

4   Propst LR (1988) *Psychotherapy in a Religious Framework*. Human Sciences Press, New York, NY, p.28.

5   This list of blocking activities is based on the blocks to listening in McKay M, Davis M and Fanning P (1983) *Messages: the communication book*. New Harbinger Publications, Oakland, CA, pp.16–19.

6   This activity is adapted from a survey found in McKay M, Davis M and Fanning P (1983) *Messages: the communication book*. New Harbinger Publications, Oakland, CA, pp.16–19.

7   McKay M, Davis M and Fanning P (1983) *Messages: the communication book*. New Harbinger Publications, Oakland, CA, p.24.

8   Pulchalski CM and Romer AL (2000) Taking a spiritual history allows clinicians to understand patients more fully. *Journal of Palliative Medicine*. **3**: 129–37.

9   Anadarajah G and Hight E (2001) Spirituality and medical practice: using the HOPE questions as a practical tool for spiritual assessment. *American Family Physician*. **63**(January 1): 1.

10 Kristeller JL and Rhodes M (2002) The OASIS Project: oncologist-assisted spirituality intervention study. Presented at *Spirituality and Health Care*. Salt Lake City, UT, March.

11 ASPIN: Assisted Spiritual Intervention. For more information contact Jean L Kristeller, PhD. pykris@scifac.indstate.edu.

12 McCullouch J, Ramesar S and Peterson H (1998) Psychotherapy in primary care: the BATHE technique. *American Family Physician*. **57**(May 1): 9.

CHAPTER 8

Spiritual assessment

> We are fragmented into so many different aspects. We don't know who we really are, or what aspects of ourselves we should identify with or believe in. So many contradictory voices, dictates, and feelings fight for control over our inner lives that we find ourselves scattered everywhere, in all directions, leaving nobody at home.
>
> Sogyal Rinpoche, *The Tibetan Book of Living and Dying*

In the preceding chapters we have explored the concept of personhood and have affirmed that each of us is a complex being that cannot be defined by the physical alone. We have examined spirituality and religion and considered how these powerful realities impact all of life. We have recognized that each person is shaped by myriad influences, and thus represents a 'culture of one.' This unique personal culture also includes a distinctive spiritual culture. Finally we have looked at the importance of clinicians and patients working together to unravel these complexities and come to an understanding of the factors which are affecting a person's ability to prevent illness, cope with illness or adversity, or access healing.

The context of spiritual assessment

The key to this process of working together is the narrative interaction between the healer and patient that develops over the course of several visits. It involves the physician, nurse, or other professional using specific tools (*see* Chapter 7) that help the patient to say what needs to be said and help the healer to better understand the patient. By facilitating this process, the healthcare professional attends to the various facets of the person's being, focusing on those that may be central to the problem.

This concept has been referred to as contextual care. Contextual care is a systems approach to healthcare that involves an expansive search for a 'context for the patient's problem that will allow the problem to be understood by both the doctor and patient and for its meaning to be explored.'[1] Possible contexts, according to this model, include biomedical, psychological, family, community, and social. A key context is the individual patient context. In the *Textbook of Family Medicine*, this individual patient context is seen to involve a wide spectrum of issues:

> What issues should be considered in the *individual patient context*? What is the patient's lifestyle? Does he or she follow any special diet or exercise plan? Does the patient consider himself or herself to be happy or satisfied with life? Is the patient able to perform the daily functions of day-to-day life? What are the patient's spiritual beliefs and how do these

affect his or her health? Each of these questions addresses not the biomedical or psychological context but the patient's life overall in an increasingly holistic context. A wise physician once said that there is no ICD-9 code for unhappiness, but an unhappy or lonely patient certainly seeks medical care more frequently than a happy one.[2]

Any look at the integration of healthcare and spirituality is best understood within a framework such as that provided by contextual care. Integration begins with the recognition that the individual patient context is important, and that one of the key elements of that context is spirituality. With integration we use specific tools, such as active listening or the BATHE technique, to expose issues that must be considered. If clues emerge that there are spiritual issues to be considered, then a process of assessment must occur that will allow the healer to develop an appropriate response, a response that is crafted and implemented in partnership with the patient.

Recognizing that physicians are not normally 'spiritual specialists' or mental health therapists, and that the clinic encounter is clearly time-limited, what are some approaches or models that might prove useful? The first thing to remember is that any assessment or 'diagnosis' needs to be made within the context of a therapeutic relationship. This means the process cannot be rushed. An overly aggressive assessment process or an assessment process that begins too early can undermine trust and destroy the sense of safety necessary for a person to reveal material that comes from the center of their being. In addition, a movement to assessment and intervention that occurs too early may result in the wrong issues being addressed. People often introduce safer, less intense issues first, moving to the most intense and most critical only gradually. Thus the first rule for effective assessment is 'take your time.' It is important to allow the therapeutic relationship to develop, probably over a series of clinical sessions. There are some who struggle with the concept of letting the process emerge progressively. First, they point out, some patients do not return on a regular basis or, because of the clinical or system infrastructure, do not experience continuity of care. This is a difficulty that cannot be ignored and is a reminder that integration of spirituality and healthcare may not be possible or appropriate in all situations. If the relationship between the clinician and patient does not involve interpersonal continuity and thus does not allow for the development of trust, integration may be unsuitable and risky. Other concerns include the fear that the issues exposed may be beyond the physician's sphere of competence or that issues may be revealed that cannot be resolved within a primary care context. Many feel uncomfortable opening up issues and discovering emotional or spiritual dis-ease if it is unlikely that substantive progress can occur within what they consider a reasonable time frame.[3] Others are concerned about the tentative nature of any assessment that involves the emotional, relational, or spiritual realms.

In response to these concerns we affirm again that assessment is an ongoing process. A clear understanding of the issues may take time to evolve, and understanding may change frequently. Not only will the healer's perception change as more information is uncovered, but patients change over time. Indeed, to hang on to an initial perception and not be open to change is a 'blocking' activity. It is also important to affirm that assessments, like interventions, should often be collaborative in nature. Just as healthcare professionals can turn to people with other specialties for help in assessing and treating a physical issue, so they can turn to spiritual specialists for help in assessing and treating spiritual issues. Psychologists, psychotherapists, religious leaders, hospital chaplains, and others can be consulted as part of the process.

The assessment itself fits into a progression that, whether it occurs in one session or spans a series of sessions, has six stages.[4] At each stage the clinician may be addressing not only the physical disease but also the spiritual dis-ease, which together create the person's state of illness. The first stage involves connecting with the patient. It is always important to create rapport with the patient, or re-establish rapport established at an earlier session. Since, when dealing with powerful issues such as anger, hopelessness, and guilt, trust is critical, this step must not be ignored. Clinicians should introduce themselves and seek to establish a connection through words, tone, and body language. Information about the healthcare professional, including name and qualifications, should be offered. A handshake, a smile, good eye contact, or other non-verbal signals can be very important in helping patients feel safe. A doctor or nurse who sits down so as to be at the same level as the patient is also helping to create a therapeutic bond. These suggestions may seem obvious, but such small initial steps are all too frequently forgotten in the midst of a busy day. It is also important to take some time to negotiate the purpose of the encounter. Patients should be asked questions that establish their understanding regarding the session and provide them with an opportunity to share what they want to achieve, their goals and expectations for the session. It is possible at this time to negotiate some small achievable goals for the session. For example, the clinician might ask the following question: 'If there is one thing you would like to achieve from our time together today, what might it be?' The answer may be predictable, but there are often surprises.

The second stage involves gathering and offering information. This will happen throughout the session in many different ways. Information will arrive through words, tone, and body language. It may come directly and indirectly. It may be overt or well hidden in clues. If the healthcare professional is open and listens carefully, the information will probably suggest one or more contexts as primary concerns to the patient. It is possible for the doctor, nurse, or other provider to control the discussion to such a degree that the patient is forced to focus on the physical realm alone. This mistake, perhaps the most common in American clinical medicine, results in a reductionist assessment of patients' problems. If the doctor, nurse, or counselor uses good listening skills and takes the time to do this step properly then misinformation, misunderstanding, and shallowness can be avoided. The goal here is to identify those context(s) for the patient's problem that allow the clearest formulation of a management plan. This step should not involve probing or coercion. Care must be taken to proceed at the patient's pace.

During the third stage the original information is explored more deeply and concerns, beliefs, and issues clarified and identified. Again, the use of active listening is critical. The use of creative questions, perception checks, and other such tools will be necessary to enable this process. What is the patient's belief about their illness? What does it mean to them? What do they believe is wrong? Why do they believe they are ill? How is their illness affecting them personally? How it is affecting their emotions and relationships? Is there any spiritual dis-ease?

The fourth stage, which occurs only after these initial steps are taken, involves the task of assessment. The assessment should be based on what has been seen, heard, and felt. It should involve the emotional, relational, physical, and spiritual facets of the person. It should be appropriately contextualized.

The fifth stage involves decisions about how to respond or intervene with respect to the most critical issues. As part of this process the physician, nurse, or counselor should summarize their perception of the issues and priorities that have been discussed. With any intense spiritual encounter the risk of error is large and it is necessary to check, re-check, and check again. The skill of paraphrase can be very helpful at this point. For example:

> **Physician**: From what I've heard and seen today you seem to have some strong feelings of guilt (spiritual issue) about your illness. Although you have some strong friendships, you are still hesitant to talk with you friends about your illness. Why is this?
> **Patient:** Yes. My church feels very strongly about taking care of the body, which is the temple of God. My smoking has always made me feel guilty and I have hidden it from my friends. I'm afraid if they know of my sickness and its connection to my behavior, they will think poorly of me and reject me.
> **Physician**: OK, I understand that you feel guilt, and that you are concerned about being rejected, let's explore how we might work with these issues...

The sixth and final stage involves establishing what follow-up there will be. Will there be another visit? What will the patient do between this session and the next? What will the healthcare professional do between this session and the next? If this is a final visit, at least for the moment, and there will be no follow-up, this should also be clarified. Even if there are no plans for another visit, patients should always be left with the feeling that help will always be available should they need it.

The assessment stage, as practiced by social workers, psychotherapists/counselors, and religious leaders, has fairly standard components. Normally an assessment addresses the presentation of the patient, a patient problem description, a psycho-socialspiritual history, a mental status exam (addressing cognition, affect, and behavior), and an impression of the clients' issues. This process closely parallels the assessment process practiced by doctors and nurses when exploring physical issues. The typical medical process includes a history of present illness from the patient, a past medical history, social history, family history, review of systems, and physical examination, perhaps including a mental status exam allowing the clinician to follow the patient's lead as the story unfolds. Consider the following example of how this might take place.

> **Physician:** Good afternoon Mrs. Smith. How can I help you today?
> **Mrs. Smith**: I'm not sure, doctor. I've been having trouble sleeping even though I feel tired all of the time. I've also been having headaches more often and have been missing work. My husband finally insisted that I see the doctor to get to the bottom of this.
> **Physician:** I can see why you're concerned. Please start at the beginning of these symptoms and tell me as much as you can about them.
> **Mrs. Smith:** Well, it's been really difficult for me since last Christmas. My mother is in poor health and I've been very worried about her. She came for a visit at Christmas time and I was shocked at how weak and

tired she was. My mother and my husband have never gotten along very well. He thinks I worry too much. But mother lives alone and she lives too far away for me to look in on her regularly. I just can't stop thinking about the story of Ruth from the bible. I really want to be a faithful daughter and to be at my mother's side. She has not had an easy life. But I have a job and a family here and can't just abandon them to care for her. I've been worrying about this almost every day and I lay awake thinking about it at night. But I am also concerned about my blood pressure, which has been higher than usual even though I take my medicine every day. Do you think I might have anemia? My appetite hasn't been good.
Physician: There are lots of medical problems that can cause fatigue, and we can certainly look into your physical health. But I'm also concerned about how worried you are about your mother. You know, that much worry can weigh heavily on someone.

This example is consistent with a contextual approach to healthcare. The physician follows the patient and is clearly thinking more broadly than physical illnesses in assessing the patient's condition. Contextual care is much more complex than simply choosing among several contexts when evaluating patients. In fact, all of the contexts are important. Medical problems like hypertension and anemia are important to assess. But so are those family, social, and spiritual issues that bother patients. It is the act of eliciting this information and using it to develop an impression of the client's spiritual issues with which we are now concerned.

In short any assessment should consider all the dimensions of self, physical, relational, emotional, and spiritual. The assessment should also include the various contexts such as biomedical, psychological, family, community and social, and individual. Keeping both dimensions and context in mind, the provider should seek to recognize clues that spiritual issues are present and find a meaningful way to think about the spiritual culture of the patient. Only in this way can one move to the next step in the process, that of meaningful intervention.

Questions for reflection

- Is a spiritual assessment indicated for all people?
- What might be the signs or clues that such an assessment is indicated?

Tools for spiritual assessment

We have, in the previous chapter, explored how to gather information about spiritual dis-ease or distress. Now it is time to explore the next step. Just as a clinician learns how to think about and analyze the physical clues or symptoms in order to establish a diagnosis, so too the clinician must learn how to think about and analyze the spiritual clues and information presented by the patient. There are a number of tools that can be used to create understanding about what is happening with a patient spiritually, and how that is affecting the healing process. These tools provide the kind of analysis or assessment necessary to move toward change and resolution.

Universal filters

One way to reflect about the spiritual dynamics present in others is to focus on how they receive, process, and then share information about spiritual issues. Some of the most powerful work around this dynamic was done by Richard Bandler and John Grinder in the mid-1970s. These two men identified what is now known as neuro-linguistic programming.[5] In a recent book on effective medical encounters, Lewis Walker, a Scottish physician, describes neuro-linguistic programming in this way:

> The *neuro* aspect is all about the mind, and how it takes in and processes information... Once inside, it passes through our various *internal filters*, such as our beliefs, values, memories, and life experiences among other things.
>
> The *linguistic* element is all about how we use our language, how we label things, how we interpret things, and how we talk, both with others *and* with ourselves.
>
> *Programming* is a word left over from the early days of the personal computer... Patterning might be a better word. Having taken in outside information (*neuro*), talked to ourselves or others about what to do (*linguistic*), we then run a series of actions or behaviors designed to achieve our particular goal in that situation (*programming*).[6]

Filtering is a critical concept of neuro-linguistic programming. We have talked a lot about the filtering process involved in receiving information (Chapter 5) and have explored some specific filters that are part our own unique histories. Bandler and Grinder identified three filtering processes that are universal. We all use these, both when we receive information and when we share it. The first of these is deletion. With deletion we simply filter out most of the pieces of information that assail us every moment of our lives. As Walker notes, 'about two million pieces of information bombard our nervous system every second. Yet we can only be consciously aware of about seven pieces at one time. We have deleted the rest.'[7] What we delete, both in terms of what we receive and what we share, may be an important clue about what is going on inside. It may in fact be the key to whatever is hindering a person in terms of creative change. Bandler and Grinder suggest that what people delete or omit from their verbal transactions is critical and might need to be 'challenged' or explored.[8] If a person simply says, 'I am struggling,' the obvious deletion relates to what the struggle is all about. What is the focus of the inner battle that is being waged? 'I am struggling with my use of alcohol' would be more complete and useful from a therapeutic standpoint.

Another key filtering process is *distortion*. The 'process of distortion involves giving labels to our experiences so that we can interpret them, make meanings out of them, evaluate them and even judge them.'[9] Distortion may involve making a process that is ongoing into an event,[10] or interpreting an event to fit with beliefs or values.[11] A person who may be struggling with a lifestyle choice in an ongoing manner may talk about the choice as if it has already been made. 'I erred when I made that decision.' In reality that person may be in the process of moving toward a certain decision, and there are still choices to be made. Another may talk about an event in a way that shows they have already made a judgment about that event or behavior, based on internal and subjective criteria. These kinds of distortions are, again, a clue and deserve reflection and perhaps attention. By being aware of these distortions we often can gain understanding about major spiritual issues that are impacting people's lives.

The final filtering process is *generalization*.[12] With generalization there is a movement away from the specific and well-defined to the vague and general. The end result is that the information that emerges is unclear and unfocused. Bandler and Grinder use the following example:

> **Client**: I'm scared
> **Therapist**: Of what?
> **Client**: Of people.

The client in this transaction is clearly being protective. It is likely that they are not scared of 'people' as much as they are afraid of a 'person.' Again, the use of this generalization filter can be seen as a clue that there is something important attached to this statement.

When any of these filters appear the listener has three options. One can simply accept what has been given, the 'impoverished model,' the distortion, or the lack of focus. Obviously the use of the filter is noted, but no overt response is made. A second option is to ask for the missing piece, or ask a question that demands more focus. In the case of 'distortions' the questions can seek to reconnect the speaker with the issues and processes involved. In short, the listener takes the free information offered by the speaker, pays attention to the clues, and asks for more information. The final option is for the clinician to make a guess, based on experience, intuition, context, and other factors, about the nature of a person's dis-ease. Normally, since such guesses are fraught with danger, these guesses must be confirmed by the use of a tool such as a perception check.

No matter which option is chosen, it is clear how focusing on these three filters can move the practitioner forward in the process of understanding the spiritual dynamics present in the patient.

Questions for reflection

- Think of a time when you have 'deleted' important information. What was the feeling attached to the information you deleted?
- Think of a time when you moved to the level of generalization. Why did you generalize rather than be specific?
- Can you remember a time when you distorted information in your communication with another? What was the significance of that distortion. Example: Why did you express a decision as completed when it was really in process? Why did you frame an event the way you did (load it with ethical implications or judgments)?
- What have you learned about yourself and your issues from reflecting on these filters?

Spiritual and religious changes

In 1995 the American Psychiatric Association developed a new category in the *Diagnostic and Statistical Manual of Mental Disorders* (DSM-IV, V62.89) for religious/spiritual problems. The purpose of this new diagnostic category was to allow clinicians to classify certain problems as uniquely spiritual or religious. The presence of this category emphasizes the fact that these kinds of problems can exist independently of other mental and/or emotional disorders. Previously spiritual issues were seen primarily as pathological symptoms. It is of course important to separate those people who have purely spiritual dis-ease from those who have mental health problems. An article in the *American Journal of Psychotherapy* provides an excellent set of guidelines for making distinction between spiritual problems and thought disorders.[13]

- Psychotic experiences are typically more intense than spiritual experiences.
- Psychotic experiences are typically ego-dystonic and are consistently terrifying to the individual, whereas religious/spiritual experiences – though uncomfortable at times – have ego-syntonic elements and frequently offer some degree of comfort to the individual.
- Psychotic experiences are often associated with a progressive deterioration in self-care.
- Psychotic experiences often involve special messages from religious figures unverified by communities of esoteric practitioners within the given tradition.
- Spiritual experiences are usually associated with good pre-episodic functioning, whereas pathology is less often associated with good pre-episode functioning.
- In psychopathology there is usually a slower onset of symptoms when there are more stressful precipitants.
- In spiritual issues, there is usually a positive explanatory attitude toward the experience.

When the problem is a matter of spiritual stress, rather than psychoses, then the clinician can begin to explore the sources of the dis-ease. We have seen how the exploration can involve something as basic as universal filters. However, the evaluative process can also focus on some very specific and well-defined issues. Some of those problems can be primarily religious, emerging from religious practice or participation in a religious system.

One possible dynamic to look for is a change in *religious orientation*. Many people who are struggling spiritually respond to their dis-ease by changing or redefining their religious affiliation. In some cases this change may involve a move within a specific faith system. There are many levels of intensity possible here. Table 8.1 opposite illustrates some possible moves within the Christian faith, ranging from low-intensity to high-intensity changes.

Changes can also take place when a person moves from one faith system to another. An example would be a person raised in the Christian faith who at some point converts to Buddhism or Islam. Other changes might involve a person with no religious background at all moving into a defined system of faith or a person moving from a spiritual framework that involves organized religion to one that is totally focused on personal spiritual practices. Such changes may well reflect spiritual hunger, with the person struggling spiritually believing that their current affiliation is not meeting their spiritual needs and seeking relief by a change of

Table 8.1 Changes in religious orientation

	Old system	New system	Dynamics
Lower intensity	Presbyterian	Presbyterian	Same denomination. Motivation often personal, including pastor, location, conflict.
	Presbyterian	Methodist	Similar denominations. Motivation normally personal.
⇕	Baptist	Presbyterian	Significantly different denominations, both Protestant. Motivation may involve values, beliefs, attitudes.
	Methodist	Roman Catholic	Different denominations, Protestant to Catholic. Motivation may involve values, beliefs, attitudes.
Higher intensity	Pentecostal holiness	Episcopalian	Different denominations. Conservative to liberal, experiential to liturgical. Motivation often spiritual hunger or crisis.

system. By noting the change we may be able to uncover a sense of spiritual emptiness. In another case it may reflect discontent with specific spiritual beliefs. People often reach a point in their spiritual journey where they are no longer comfortable with 'old truths.' They find themselves unable to adhere to certain doctrines and thus must change their religious affiliation. For others the change is simply an emotional response to a negative experience, one that may be recent or in the distant past. In some cases the change may not be voluntary, but forced. A person who is coerced into a specific faith system by marriage may become angry and alienated. It used to be mandatory for people marrying a Roman Catholic to become Catholic themselves. At the very least, people were asked to guarantee that they would raise their children according to that faith system. In some cases this forced movement into a strange and sometimes uncomfortable system creates spiritual stress. It must be noted that such changes are not indicative of spiritual distress alone. People will also make such changes as the result of a deep and positive spiritual experience. A change may be a sign of spiritual awakening or rebirth. It may reflect a conversion experience, or a powerful experience of the divine. Even a 'forced' change may be a joyful and positive event, reflective of a positive event, a marriage or the birth of a child, in a person's life. Part of the assessment process should include not only an examination of current religious affiliation, but an exploration of a person's spiritual history. Have there been changes in religious or spiritual orientation? What was the catalyst for change?

Sometimes the change will not be that of spiritual orientation, but *of religious or spiritual intensity*. The person's faith system doesn't change, but the way they practice faith does. Frequently when people have an intense spiritual experience, either positive or negative, it will be reflected by increased or decreased spiritual activity. A person who was once active in public worship on a regular basis may suddenly stop attending church. Indeed, a change in worship patterns is one of the most reliable indications of spiritual distress. It is almost always indicative, no matter what the stated reason, of spiritual anxiety. Another person may begin reading spiritual writings, or begin to pray or meditate on a regular basis. Another person might begin to adhere more closely to the behavioral norms of their particular faith system, such as abstinence from alcohol use. Part of the assessment process should thus include not only an exploration of current religious practice, but also changes of intensity in that practice. Has there been a change? What has caused this change? A powerful spiritual experience? Guilt? Trauma?

Questions for reflection

- Have you ever had a significant change in your spiritual or religious affiliation or practices?
- What was the event or situation that was the catalyst for this change?
- What were the feelings attached to the event or situation?

Troubling beliefs

It is always a bit dangerous to move from looking at process to looking at content when it comes to spiritual health. What seems healthy to one faith system or one person may seem unhealthy to another. Some faith systems have values and beliefs that are rejected by others. Some people may find a belief comforting, which for others creates great distress. So great care must be taken when making a judgment about the content of a person's faith. However, it is possible to see a person in spiritual distress and follow that distress back to a specific belief and label that belief as troublesome, at least for that person. Again, we must reinforce that it is possible that a specific belief which is toxic for one person may be benign, even beneficial for another. What makes a belief troubling is how it impacts the person. Does it create distress? Does it hinder recovery? Is it something they have difficulty resolving?

This being said, it seems clear there are some beliefs that frequently create spiritual distress. Just as a clinician faced with specific symptoms in a patient might look for causes normally associated with those symptoms, so a clinician when faced with spiritual symptoms can screen for these specific problematic beliefs. Listed below are some of those beliefs.

- **Faith equals healing:** Many people have the belief, to one degree or another, that God, the divine, or the sacred has a role in the healing process. This can be a very healthy belief and can provide people with a great deal of comfort and hope. However, this belief can be problematic and create spiritual distress if a couple of dynamics are present. The first issue has to do with the person's definition of healing. For many people the concept of healing is broad and includes relational, spiritual, and emotional healing as well as physical. However, some people narrow the concept of healing down to physical cure. When this happens, and they seek healing through their religion or spirituality, and it doesn't happen, they can become angry, feel disconnected from the divine, and move into hopelessness. Another issue has to do with the notion that the result is directly connected to the quality or depth of faith. People may believe, or may be told, that if they have enough faith, healing is guaranteed. One patient who was very despondent about a treatable cancer, and non-compliant in terms of her treatment plan, was found to be stuck in a state of hopelessness because she was not able to make her illness disappear through prayer. She saw her poor health as an indictment of her faith.

- **Faith as prophylactic:** Another version of the belief that faith will bring healing is the belief that the person who has a good relationship with the divine, or is walking in 'the way' will be blessed – will receive blessings, including monetary success, and will avoid major illness or disappointment. Even the most spiritual of people experience failure, illness, and disappointment. When people with this belief encounter difficulties they often experience dis-ease. What does one do when the 'formula' doesn't work? In response to this harsh reality some people choose to believe negative things about the sacred God, the divine; whatever they feel connected to has betrayed them, is capricious, or perhaps powerless. Others choose to believe negative things about themselves, specifically about their faith, which they perceive to be insufficient. Either way this group can present with hopelessness, guilt, anger, even fear. Life is very frightening when God seems unreliable and faith proves inadequate. Such people become isolated, uncooperative, and depressed.
- **Illness equals 'sin':** Many people adhere to the idea that sin, wrong actions, or error leads to illness. This idea is related to the concept that faithfulness will lead to health. With this belief, however, the focus is on the negative and causality moves backwards from whatever plagues the person to some attitude or behavior that they consider negative, perhaps even evil. The person who sees their lung cancer as related to their smoking may be correct. But it becomes toxic when it is spiritualized. In these instances the idea that smoking caused the cancer is transformed into the belief that the cancer is a punishment for smoking. There is an important difference between these two perceptions. This mentality is one that images a punitive God and creates blame and shame. With this mentality, patients move from regret (for the smoking) to guilt, perhaps even shame. The ability of the sacred to be a resource is minimized by such a causal role. The belief becomes even more toxic when the causal connection is tenuous or neurotic. The belief that an illness was caused by infidelity, untruthfulness, or a failure to adhere to religious rules can create significant spiritual distress. Again, patients find themselves mired in the realm of the negative, and spirituality instead of being a healing resource becomes a barrier to progress.
- **Faith equals passivity:** Faith in the divine can be a wonderful thing, offering many positive benefits. For most people their dominant concept is that God, or however one envisions the sacred, is a positive power. The sacred is a resource that can be accessed as one works to make the most out of life. One can rely on the divine. In the Christian religion, for example, many people see God as a partner who will work with them to maximize life and, when illness is present, will work with them and others (including healthcare professionals) to create healing. The problem comes when belief in the power of the sacred causes people to abrogate their own personal responsibility. Instead of investing any personal energy into the process of healing they simply wait for God to do whatever needs to be done. If nothing happens, then it is not 'God's will.' People with this view often use phrases such as 'It's all in God's hands' and 'Whatever God wills,' while at the same time avoiding action. Such people may violate treatment plans, ignore diets, fail to take medications, and continue unhealthy behaviors. They tend to

sink into a state of helplessness, believing that what they do will not affect or determine the outcome.

- **Authority equals mandate:** Another problem belief is that one must always submit to spiritually ordained authority. In some cases this authority is religious or spiritual leaders, and in other cases it is authorities defined by the religious system. Such authorities may include the government, group leaders, parents, or even spouses. One problem is that in accepting such radical submission, people lose the ability to make their own decisions. This problem is exacerbated by the fact that such authorities are not always beneficial, or even benign. Letting another make your decisions is made worse when that person is abusive, controlling, or selfish. This belief can lead people into situations that are devastating, involving physical and mental abuse, and can minimize them as people. A wife who must do whatever her husband says is vulnerable to such abuse, as are children when parents assume decision-making authority. Men, women, and even entire families may find themselves damaged when religious leaders become controlling. People can end up in financial difficulties, be forced to change jobs, and even be asked to move physically to a specific location. When this kind of control is present it becomes a difficulty for the clinician. Wives must get permission to adhere to a treatment plan, and may be prevented from compliance. Abuse may be accepted and thus not reported. Unhealthy behaviors, such as an inadequate diet, may be continued. This conflict with spiritual belief has become a common concern in caring for women in fundamentalist faith systems. Such conflicts between respecting spiritual beliefs and protecting patients are among the most confounding moral conflicts healthcare providers can encounter.

- **All is from God:** One book calls this mentality 'the Pollyanna Perspective.'[14] This is the belief that everything that happens is from God and thus everything that happens is purposeful and appropriate. Not necessarily comfortable or positive from a 'worldly' perspective, but appropriate. The problem with this perspective is that it does not allow for life's polarities. Sometimes it is appropriate to say, 'this is bad' or 'this needs to change.' But with this point of view all that happens is part of a divine plan. It is not appropriate then to experience the sadness, anger, or helplessness that normally result from negative events. With this belief people not only fail to look realistically at the bad elements present in their lives, but they avoid dealing with the destructive feelings that afflict them. Again, some people may find comfort in this concept, and even use this idea to resolve their feelings about illness. But in other cases resolution doesn't come and anger and disappointment begin to dominate.

- **Suffering servant:** This belief is founded upon the idea that one can and must 'serve' or 'work' one's way into spiritual fulfillment, enlightenment, or heaven. Certainly the idea of promoting good and serving others is usually healthy. However, at times this belief can reach an extreme level, causing the person to neglect their own needs and health. In one instance a patient was suffering from a variety of physical ailments. She was afflicted by arthritis in her back and hips. She had respiratory issues that left her short of breath and with low oxygen levels in her blood. She was often tired. Finally her health deteriorated until she was losing weight and was becoming increasingly frail. In spite of these difficulties and the fact that she worked part time, she spent a significant amount of time caring for her grandchildren. Although her daughter was capable of watching the children, this woman saw providing this service as her duty and would not lessen her efforts. In some cases this kind of belief can lead to what is essentially a 'personal martyr complex'[15] and may cause people to be intentionally self-destructive. The more their 'service' costs them, the more spiritual they feel.

This list of religious problems is certainly not inclusive, but does illustrate the kind of issues that may contribute to illness or be a hindrance to healing. Many of these issues emerge from beliefs that are not inherently problematic. In most cases the problems come when the beliefs are carried to extremes, or when the polarities of life are ignored and balance is lost. Wanting to serve is good, wanting to serve to the point that one's health is compromised is not. Believing that good things come from one's connection to the divine is good. Believing that nothing 'bad' can happen when one has a relationship to the divine is not. A balanced view might accept the benefit of a relationship with the divine and an understanding that bad things can happen. In such a case spirituality does not make us impervious to negative events, but provides us with important resources when such events do unfold.

We must look for religious beliefs that worsen people's distress, focusing not so much on the content of these beliefs as the impact of these beliefs. Clinicians may well unveil beliefs with which they personally are uncomfortable, but which do not appear to create difficulties for the patient. These kinds of beliefs should be noted, but should not be the focus of the assessment. The critical beliefs are those that create obstructive spiritual thinking and contribute to physical, relational, emotional, or spiritual problems.

Questions for reflection

- Have you ever encountered a spiritual belief that was contributing or causing physical, spiritual, emotional, or relational problems in a person?
- What was that belief?
- How did you respond to that belief?

Spiritual inventories

In some cases clinicians may want to use spiritual inventories that have been created to help assess spiritual wellness. It may not be possible for these kinds of surveys to be used extensively in the primary care setting. The most frequent use of these inventories will be by mental health or religious/spiritual professionals. However, there may be some clinicians who choose to use such tools in indicated situations. An initial spiritual assessment, using active listening skills, may point to the realm of the spiritual as a potential source of difficulties. In such cases an inventory might be used to determine the most appropriate course of action.

The measurement tools available are numerous.[16] However, many of them are designed more for research purposes than for clinical application. Many of the inventories focus on aspects of religiosity since religious practices are much easier to measure than subjective spirituality. These measures look at belief, affiliation, activity, and commitment. Many of them are focused on specific religious systems, such as Christianity, Judaism, Islam, and Buddhism. It is unlikely that most of these measures would be useful to the clinician.

Other measures are designed to explore a broad spectrum of religious, spiritual, and psychological factors rather than religiosity alone. Among this group are some measures that are accessible and brief enough for clinical application. The *Spiritual Well-Being Scale* was presented by Ellison in 1983.[17] One of the valuable aspects of this scale is the fact that it explores both people's religiosity and more generalized spiritual states. This 20-question tool consists of a 10-item religious well-being scale and a 10-item scale focus on existential issues.

The *Index of Core Spiritual Experiences* is a seven-item scale that focuses on spiritual experiences and seeks to measure feelings related to God's existence, closeness to God, and a sense of God' presence within.[18] It was originally used to assess adults with serious and chronic medical problems, including chronic pain, hypertension, and cancer. The key descriptor for the sacred in this scale is God, which allows it to embrace a broader definition of spirituality than many measures. It would not be as useful for people with a faith orientation rooted in eastern religions.

The *Spiritual Wellness Inventory* was developed by Ingersoll in 1995.[19] This inventory is based upon a set of 10 spiritual dimensions, including conception of the absolute/divine, meaning, connectedness, mystery, spiritual freedom, experience/ritual, forgiveness, hope, knowledge/learning, and present-centeredness. It was designed to be used as a starting point for dialogue with the patient about spiritual issues. Because it is broken into dimensions it allows problem areas to emerge quickly. For example, if the scores across dimensions are fairly consistent, but the 'connectedness' dimension is significantly lower, then this provides a point of focus. The patient can be asked to comment on why they believe this particular score is so irregular. This inventory is not short, consisting of 55 questions, but has the advantage of a provocative scoring system.

The *Spiritual Involvement and Beliefs Scale* was developed by a primary care physician. This scale involves 22 questions designed to examine both the spiritual beliefs and religious practices of patients. It is short and very appropriate for use in the clinical setting.[20] You can find the latest version of this scale in Appendix B.

Some clinicians who regularly integrate medicine and spirituality develop a preference for specific scales and use them regularly in their work with patients. In some cases the scale is used universally. In other cases the scale is used for indicated or selected patient populations. When used universally, the survey is given to all or most patients during the process of obtaining a medical history. In most cases, however, such an instrument is used with either selective or indicated groups. A selective group would be comprised of those patients who are at risk for spiritual distress. An example of a patient who would fall into this category would be one whose illness had potential moral overtones, such as a sexually transmitted disease or HIV/AIDS. Another example might be a patient with a chronic or terminal illness. An indicated group might be those who have shown signs that they are struggling in the spiritual dimension. A patient from this group would be a person who offers a clear clue during a clinical session that they are struggling with guilt or hopelessness.

We suggest that such tools be used not to define the spiritual health of the patient, but to provide, as Ingersoll suggests, a starting point for dialogue. Ultimately any spiritual assessment should be a collaborative process involving both the clinician and patient. Conclusions should be negotiated and agreed upon by both parties.

Hatch's belief scale is included in Appendix B. Dr Ingersoll's tool is available at the back of *Explorations in Spirituality and Counseling* (Faiver *et al.*).[15] Information regarding the other scales can be found in the *Handbook of Religion and Health* (Koenig, McCullough and Larson).[16]

The spiritual issues spectrum

The collaborative nature of the assessment process is the key to using the Spiritual Issues Spectrum. This spectrum, which was introduced in Chapter 4, takes some key spiritual issues and establishes a set of polarities. This spectrum not only helps illustrate the impact, both positive and negative, of spirituality, but can serve as an excellent assessment tool. The spectrum is based upon words we have found meaningful. However, this spectrum is not inviolate and can be adjusted to meet personal needs. Not everyone uses the same terminology, and it is entirely appropriate for a clinician to develop a set of spectrums using their own personal terminology.

The spectrum can be effectively used to think about the spiritual status of an individual patient and provide an excellent foundation for planning appropriate interventions. We will illustrate the use of the spectrum by using the case of Anne.

Anne was a 34-year-old female, married and with one 5-year-old child. Anne presented at her primary care clinic with undifferentiated abdominal pain. The physician was unable to identify a clear cause for Anne's pain, but suggested it might be irritable bowel syndrome. He treated her symptoms with a low-dose antidepressant. Unfortunately her symptoms did not improve and she became a regular visitor to the clinic. During one of her visits Anne told a story about being lost as a child. She noted that when she was finally found her father was furious, and banished her to her bedroom for the weekend. The story was somewhat out of sync with the overall visit, so the doctor made a brief note about it in his notes. About a month later, as he explored the potential stressors contributing to her pain, the physician decided to ask the FICA questions. Anne affirmed that she believed in God (Faith) but noted that although raised in a church, she had been unable to find a church in which she felt comfortable. She affirmed that she believed faith was very important (Importance), but again, denied involvement in any community (C) of faith. When asked how her faith might apply (A) to her health she became angry and made the comment that she couldn't share her spiritual thoughts with a male. The physician used a perception check to explore her feeling state. 'Are you uncomfortable with a male physician?' She responded by noting that she was uncomfortable with all males. 'Including your husband?' 'Yes.'

Eventually the physician, meeting strong resistance, suggested Anne switch to a female physician who practiced at the same clinic. Alerted to the fact that Anne might have significant emotional, relational, or spiritual issues the physician decided to take some time to explore Anne's spiritual issues. What she eventually discovered was that Anne was a victim of sexual abuse at the hands of her father. This man was an active member of a very conservative Christian church and was very overt about his religion. He attended church regularly and participated in a bible study. He often used his religion as a justification for his actions. He was extremely controlling and dominated his wife and children with a heavy hand, demanding submission because the Bible established a 'clear chain of command.' In the family the husband was the leader and should always be obeyed. He had verbally abused his wife, Anne's mother, and she was extremely withdrawn. He often shouted at Anne and frequently hit her. When she was about nine years old, he began to fondle her and eventually had sex with her on a regular basis. He demanded secrecy and threatened not only physical harm, but eternal damnation if she told anyone about their 'relationship.'

After leaving her home Anne had tried very hard to develop a normal life. She had married and had been sexually active with her husband, although she felt very uncomfortable with any sort of sexuality. She found herself growing angry and resentful at her husband's insistence that they have sex. Struggling with feelings of anger and hopelessness, she tried to turn to the church. Unfortunately this attempt was not successful. In each Christian church, the image used to describe God was frequently that of father. She found that this caused her to transfer her anger at her father to God, and she was rarely able to make it completely through a service of worship. Intensifying matters was the fact that all of the ministers in her community were male. She found it very difficult to relate to these male authority figures, and often found herself repulsed by them for no apparent reason. She related a time that she had attempted to talk to one of the more sensitive ministers. His church was relatively careful about gender-related images for God and she found it the most comfortable. However, she soon found herself shouting at the minister, telling him she hated God and she hated him. She left without revealing the basis of her anger.

Eventually the physician was able to connect Anne with a psychotherapist who was comfortable with spiritual issues. In this safe environment Anne began to deal with the reality of her abuse and began the road to emotional, spiritual, and relational healing.

What would it look like if we related Anne's spiritual situation to the spectrum we have developed? Assuming that each spectrum represents a scale from 1 to 10, where would she fall between each of the polarities?

Despair or Hope
Helplessness or Empowerment
Anger or Forgiveness
Guilt/Curse or Restoration/Blessing
Fear or Serenity
Disconnection or Connection

The first polarity is despair and hope. If despair is a 1 and hope is a 10, where does Anne fall? Based upon the fact that Anne was actively seeking to connect with the divine it is logical to believe that there was still some degree of hope present.

Although she was doubtful about her future, she was still attempting to move forward. However, conversation with her physician also showed the potential for her to slip into despair. On this spectrum we might place her in the middle at 5.

The second polarity involves the polarities of helplessness or empowerment. Again, Anne is fairly proactive. She has sought out both medical and spiritual help and is willing to participate in psychotherapy. It is clear she does not feel totally helpless. Her participation in developing a treatment plan and her compliance reflect a reasonable degree of empowerment. Her frustration over her ability to find a spiritual home is frustrating to her and lowers her score on this spectrum slightly, but we might place her toward the empowerment pole at a 7.

The third polarity is anger and forgiveness. Anne is clearly angry. Her most intense anger is directed at her father, but that anger is spilling over into many other relationships. She has transferred that anger to most males, including her husband and any males in a position of power (including ministers and physicians). It appears that her anger has not been directed at her 5-year-old son. Ultimately her anger has become focused on the divine, who in her religious tradition is often anthropomorphized as a male, and is given the image of father. Although it is overwhelmed by her anger toward others, there is also some underlying anger at herself. She is angry that she has allowed herself to be victim and angry that she cannot resolve her problems on her own. We must place her totally on the anger pole at a 1.

Her self-anger leads naturally to the fourth polarity, which is guilt and forgiveness. Because Anne is the victim in this scenario we might tend to think that guilt would not be an issue. On this spectrum Anne did not offer many clues, but it is not unusual for the victims of abuse to have a very strong sense of guilt. They often believe that somehow the abuse is their fault, that in some manner they 'asked for' or 'deserved' what occurred. On this spectrum we would place a question mark slightly slanted toward the guilt end of the spectrum. Anne's self-anger is at least indicative that she has not forgiven herself.

The fifth polarity is fear and serenity. Fear, as we have defined it, is to some degree a matter of chaos. When in the realm of fear, one is struggling with not only the present but also the past and the future. Such people are unhappy with what has been, find their present a matter of chaos, and have no confidence about the future. Anne is clearly in turmoil. There is almost nothing about her life that feels comfortable. She is very 'raw' and, as she describes it, 'constantly waiting for the shoe to drop.' She is apprehensive and worries about when she will next lose control of her emotions. She is fearful that she will yell at her husband or her child, so fearful that her anger may overwhelm her and force her to get up and leave a service of worship. She falls on the spectrum at around a 2.

The final polarity is that of disconnection and connection. Anne feels radically disconnected from God, the church, and her husband. She finds it difficult to relate to any male. On the other hand, she does have some women friends, and is beginning to build relationships of trust with both her female physician and her psychotherapist. However, we are assessing her spiritual state, and at this point she feels not only disconnected but repelled by the male image of God that is dominant in her tradition. Because of her desire to connect with the divine we might move her to a 2. If she can begin to image the divine as feminine or in some way non-male, the sense of connectedness will likely grow.

Thus our Spiritual Spectrum for Anne might look like as shown in Figure 8.1.

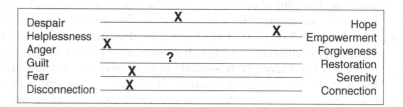

Figure 8.1

Spiritual Spectrums are often the end product of a process. Throughout the process, information is gathered using active listening skills with a focus on identifying spiritual clues. The clues are then analyzed using a variety of concepts or models. The clinician looks for universal filters, significant spiritual changes, specific spiritual problems, and finally, the spiritual themes included in the Spiritual Spectrum. All of the information is gathered, synthesized, and then used to complete the spectrum.

There is another way in which the Spiritual Spectrum can be used. Clinicians often ask patients to share their own unique perspective of their illness. They ask patients to rate pain or discomfort. 'On a scale from 1 to 10, how is your pain?' They ask patients to describe, to image their ailment. 'Describe the kind of feeling you have. Is it sharp, as if you are being stabbed with a knife, or is it more of a throbbing kind of pain?' It is entirely appropriate to ask patients to complete the spiritual spectrum themselves. It is suggested the scale not have a number, but simply consist of a line between the two poles. All the patient needs to do is place a mark that illustrates where they see themselves in terms of the polarity.

Such assessments are not an end in themselves but a tool that points toward a next step. The Spiritual Spectrum prepares the clinician to answer three basic questions.

1 Are there points of spiritual distress that may need addressing as part of the therapeutic process?
2 Are there themes or issues that need to be watched?
3 Are there positive themes that need to be supported and encouraged? Where are the strengths on which we can build?

Our analysis of the spectrum must always be contextual. The fact that a person is on what might be seen as the 'negative' end of the spectrum is not always a matter of great concern. The issue is normally this: 'Is it appropriate for this person to be at this place at this time?' If a person who has lived a healthy lifestyle has just learned they have a terminal illness normally caused by behaviors such as smoking or alcohol abuse, it is normal and predictable that they feel angry. If a person has just learned that their condition cannot be resolved by medical science, it may be very appropriate for them to feel a sense of helplessness. The spectrum merely provides a 'snapshot in time.'

The clinician's goal is to work with the patient to decide how the profile should change and how it should remain the same. In short, we move from developing an assessment to developing treatment goals, and then planning interventions that will help meet those goals. It is to the issues of outcome and interventions that we now move in the final chapter.

Questions for reflection

- If you were to develop six sets of spiritual polarities, what would they be?
- If you were to fill out a spiritual spectrum, how would it look?
- How does your spectrum reflect your life context?
- What are your spiritual strengths?
- Where would you like to see change or movement?

Notes

1   Saultz JW (1999) *Textbook of Family Medicine*. McGraw-Hill Publishers, New York, NY.
2   Saultz JW (1999) *Textbook of Family Medicine*. McGraw-Hill Publishers, New York, NY.
3   Bryant-Jefferies R (2003) *Time Limited Therapy in Primary Care*. Radcliffe Medical Press, Oxford, p.6.
4   Session components adapted from Bor R, Miller R, Latz M and Salt H (1998) *Counseling in Health Care Settings*. Cassell, New York, NY, pp.65–9.
5   Bandler R and Grinder J (1979) *frogs into PRINCES*. Real People Press, Moab, UT.
6   Walker L (2002) *Consulting with NLP: neuro-linguistic programming in the medical consultation*. Radcliffe Medical Press, Oxford, pp.16, 17.
7   Walker L (2002) *Consulting with NLP: neuro-linguistic programming in the medical consultation*. Radcliffe Medical Press, Oxford, p.17.
8   Bandler R and Grinder J (1975) *The Structure of Magic*. Science and Behavior Books, Palo Alto, CA, pp.40–3.
9   Walker L (2002) *Consulting with NLP: neuro-linguistic programming in the medical consultation*. Radcliffe Medical Press, Oxford, p.18.
10 Bandler R and Grinder J (1975) *The Structure of Magic*. Science and Behavior Books, Palo Alto, CA, p.43.
11 Walker L (2002) *Consulting with NLP: neuro-linguistic programming in the medical consultation*. Radcliffe Medical Press, Oxford, p.18.
12 Bandler R and Grinder J (1975) *The Structure of Magic*. Science and Behavior Books, Palo Alto, CA. pp.47–9.
13 Greenberg D and Witzum E (1991) Problems in the treatment of religious patients. *American Journal of Psychotherapy*. **45**: 554–64.
14 Favier C, Ingersoll RE, O'Brien E and McNally C (2001) *Explorations in Counseling and Spirituality*. Brooks/Cole (Thomson Learning), Toronto, Canada, p.100.
15 Favier C, Ingersoll RE, O'Brien E and McNally C (2001) *Explorations in Counseling and Spirituality*. Brooks/Cole (Thomson Learning), Toronto, Canada, p.100.
16 Koenig HG, McCullough ME and Larson DB (2001) *Handbook of Religion and Health*. Oxford University Press, New York, NY. Chapter 33 provides an extensive listing of current measurement tools.
17 Ellison CW (1983) Spiritual well-being: conceptualization and measurement. *Journal of Psychology and Theology*. **11**: 330–40.
18 Kass JD, Friedman R, Leserman J, Zuttermeister PC and Benson H (1991) Health outcomes and a new index of spiritual experience (INSPIRIT). *Journal for the Scientific Study of Religion*. **30**: 203–11.
19 Favier C, Ingersoll RE, O'Brien E and McNally C (2001) *Explorations in Counseling and Spirituality*. Brooks/Cole (Thomson Learning), Toronto, Canada, Appendix G, pp.185–94.
20 Hatch RL (1998) Spiritual Involvement and Beliefs Scale. *The Journal of Family Practice*. **46**(6): 485–6.

CHAPTER 9

Spiritual interventions

I don't think people should be blamed for being sick, or blame themselves for creating their sickness. But the cost of stripping illness of meaning is too high. We demean our own experience. You want to take the moralizing out of the meaning, but if you don't search for meaning, you don't become your own authority.

Gerald Epstein[1]

John was a man in his mid-fifties who had been very successful in life. He had gone through a series of prestigious careers and had consistently found himself in leadership positions. He presented to his family physician with both severe heartburn and high blood pressure. Initial treatment plans involved ranitidine for the heartburn and instructions to monitor his blood pressure and lose weight. As the relationship between the physician and John developed, he began to reveal that he had experienced a long-term struggle with addictive behavior, using a variety of 'medications' including sex, alcohol, and work. He noted that he often played a 'tape' in his head, replaying moments in which he had behaved shamefully. He noted that it was a vicious cycle. He would remember a behavior of which he was ashamed, and as a result of the feelings that engendered, he would seek to medicate. That medicating behavior often involved a new episode of which he was ashamed, adding to the library of mental tapes. He seemed to be in a pattern that trapped him and created a great deal of spiritual distress. Eventually the physician offered John a couple of options. One option was to develop a 'ritual of release.' Since John did believe in a forgiving God, each time he recalled something he believed needed forgiveness, he was to write it down, as an act of confession, and offer it to God. He could destroy the note in whatever manner he chose. The other option was to connect with a 12-step program and learn from a sponsor there how to use 'amends' as a healing tool. John chose the first option, and eventually, because of a close Roman Catholic friend, began to confess weekly to a local Roman Catholic priest. Eventually his feelings of guilt and distress began to dissipate and he found it easier to avoid destructive and hurtful behaviors.

This creative intervention addressed the spiritual condition of the patient, and the intervention, which was primarily a matter of finding options and supporting action choices, had a positive impact on both the patient's dis-ease and disease. Because the clinician was able to identify a critical spiritual issue and facilitated an intervention, the patient was able to address his guilt and decrease his physical symptoms.

Once information has been gathered and a spiritual assessment has been made, what then? We have identified a set of core objectives for the integration of medicine and spirituality. Now it is time to explore some strategies for accomplishing these objectives. What kind of interventions will help patients achieve self-awareness, explore their spiritual frameworks, and identify creative options? How far can we go, considering the amount of time available? What level of care is possible considering the spiritual and/or counseling expertise of the clinician?

Preparing for intervention
Understanding levels of intervention

The clinician can, at least to some degree, function as a counselor. This is not a concept that is foreign to many physicians who are often placed in that position by patients. Patients will frequently bring up such issues as marital stress, addiction problems, depression, anxiety, and ethical dilemmas. In one small rural community a family physician was even asked to advise a family on what college their child should attend. The question is not so much *if* the clinician should function as a type of counselor, but *at what level*?

First we must ask what we mean by the term 'counseling.' This task can potentially include a wide range of activities. It has been suggested that counseling can involve three basic functions or levels.[2] The first function is what might be called active listening. At this level the clinician uses basic listening skills to help the patient express their feelings and disclose their issues. Also, through empathic listening, the clinician is able to show compassion and express empathy. The second function is that of offering counsel. At this level clinicians take a slightly more active role by interacting with free information offered by the patient. At this level the practitioner may amplify information given by the patient, adding new, perhaps critical, knowledge. They can challenge patients by helping them see distortions, generalizations, and deletions. They can help patients to see their 'life rules' and aid in the process of affirming, adjusting, or abandoning those rules. The third function is that of psychotherapy. Psychotherapy differs from counseling in its nature, intensity, and duration. With psychotherapy the professional relationship is primarily focused on the task of removing, modifying, and decreasing symptoms related to an emotional disturbance or mental illness. In general a lack of time and training precludes most physicians from functioning at this level. However, the first two levels, those of active listening and providing counsel, are both appropriate and possible within the usual context of the healthcare setting.

Limitations

There are, clearly, limits to what the healthcare provider can offer in either the inpatient or outpatient setting. If we return to the concerns listed earlier by primary care physicians,[3] we can easily understand what some of those limits are. First, there is the issue of time. The fact that many clinical encounters are being forced into a short time frame, as little as 15 minutes, makes it difficult for the physician to interact with the patient around spiritual matters. The biomedical imperative of the visit is dominant and can preclude other issues from being discussed. However, in many cases issues do emerge, and studies have shown that addressing those issues can actually assist the biomedical agenda. A study of 116 routine office visits found that in over half of the clinical encounters the patients offered clues about issues that were troubling them. In 60% of those cases the issues were emotional in nature. If the physician picked up the clue and responded to it in a meaningful manner, the time spent with the patient tended to be shorter than when the clue was ignored.[4] If a person feels strongly enough about an issue to reveal it, even indirectly, then it may be important enough to pull the focus away from other agendas. By hearing the clue and responding to it, the clinician may free the patient to focus on the biomedical agenda. The lack of time available does not affect whether or not spiritual issues *should* be addressed, but it does impact the degree to which it *can* be addressed. Time constraints may keep the intervention to the levels of active listening and offering counsel.

Another key limitation is the lack of training received by physicians with respect to emotional or spiritual problems. Over the past 10 years, a significant number of medical schools have begun to include the topic of medicine and spirituality in their curriculum, both as elective and required elements.[5] In spite of this, most physicians have only minimal training in the art of integrating spirituality and medicine. First, this movement is relatively new, so physicians who graduated from medical school before 1995 are unlikely to have had any training at all. Second, many such courses provide students with the rationale for integration and information about major religious groups, but do not truly provide the students with the basic skills necessary to effect integration (such as active listening skills). Third, the level of training rarely enables physicians to engage in long-term, in-depth therapy. Clinicians can help with awareness and reflection, but often are not prepared to move deeply into the issue.

This combination of minimal time and negligible training means that the primary role of the physician is that of catalyst. In the clinical encounter physicians can bring spiritual issues or needs to the awareness of patients, and begin the process of helping the patients explore and resolve these issues. But ultimately resolution will come only as the process of healing continues outside the clinical context. Patients will need to use their new awareness and knowledge as a starting point for serious spiritual work. In some cases, this work may be done by the individuals themselves, through activities such as prayer, reading, or meditation. In other cases, spiritual experts can become involved in the process. Chaplains, spiritual leaders, and psychotherapists can work with the patients to help them continue the process of spiritual recovery. This does not mean that the role of the physician or nurse is unimportant. People faced with illness or death, people engaged in an environment that is strange and frightening are uniquely vulnerable. This vulnerability is both a danger and an opportunity. The danger is that patients will disintegrate in the face of such challenges. The opportunity is that the very presence of disease and dis-ease can generate openness, change, and growth. The physician can be a catalyst for growth.

Prerequisites

Before a clinician can begin to integrate spirituality into the healthcare context and introduce any sort of intervention, there are a number of prerequisites that are important to observe. The first prerequisite is for the clinician to have a clear understanding of his or her own spiritual beliefs and world view. What we believe and the values we hold, have a significant impact on how we respond to people and events.

> Peter was a young physician who joined a practice in a small rural community in eastern Washington. He truly enjoyed the small farming community and its people and found his practice rewarding. However, there was one patient he could not stand. Mel was a 69-year-old wheat farmer. He was suffering from emphysema due to a lifetime of smoking. In spite of his smoking, which he called his 'major vice,' Mel was a very religious man. He belonged to a small independent church nestled among the wheat fields about 4 miles from town. During his clinical exams Mel often sprinkled his responses with religious phrases. He talked about being 'washed in the blood of the lamb' and about the 'redeemed life.' He often made negative statements about what he considered 'unchristian' behavior. He was very confident in his own faith, and noted that when he died he'd be 'dancing on streets of gold.' Mel's illness had him close to death. Although he was coping with his situation admirably and was a compliant patient, Peter found himself repelled by Mel. His sessions with Mel were often brief and were relationally cold. Mel clearly sensed this, and after about 6 months, transferred to another clinic about 40 miles away.
>
> When Mel died, Peter attended the funeral. It was as he sat in that small church that he suddenly realized what had happened. Peter had been raised in a church very much like Mel's. When he was in grade school his mother, who was single, had become sexually active with a man. The church leaders had discovered this and had called his mother before the congregation. They rebuked her and forced her into an emotional confession of her sin, and expelled her from the fellowship. Peter had been very angry over this treatment. His mother, who eventually married her lover, simply changed churches, and became active in a small Methodist church. Peter had vowed never to attend church again, and had been as good as his word. Sitting at that funeral he realized that he had projected his anger at that childhood church on to Mel, whose words had reminded him of that church.

We must understand our own spiritual, religious, and cultural filters. In this way we can better understand our responses to those we work with and ensure that they are healthy and appropriate. The Family Practice Residency Program at Oregon Health and Science University in Portland, Oregon, includes a curriculum on the integration of medicine and spirituality. As part of that curriculum faculty members encourage young physicians to explore their own spirituality by using the journey model. They ask the learners to think back on their spiritual history. What were some of the key moments along the way? What impact did these key moments have? How did they affect the journey? The educational goal is to help the learners understand where they are at this point in their own journeys. Students have illustrated their journeys in many ways. Some have drawn spiritual 'maps,' others have brought in pictures illustrating key moments in the journey, or written a narrative. For many of them it has been the first time, or the first time in many years, that they have thought about their spiritual life and journey. The exercise not only helps them explore the past, but it helps them begin to define their hopes for the future. Clinicians can also use one of the spiritual assessment tools that are available. The strategy for gaining self-awareness is not critical, but the act of gaining that awareness is.

Second, it is important for any person using spiritual interventions to have some degree of spiritual accountability. One physician in Portland uses her local rabbi as a spiritual supervisor or consultant. In the context of this relationship she explores spiritual issues and examines her own responses. Groups can also serve this purpose. Balint or professional support groups, for example, allow clinicians the opportunity to explore the psychological or spiritual aspects of their patients' problems – and reflect upon the way they are interacting with their patients.[6] Supervision or study groups, in which the spiritual issues that come to light through the therapeutic alliance can be further explored, have been recommended by Fukuyama and Sevig,[7] experts in the integration of spirituality and counseling.

Ideally, those who would address spiritual issues in practice should be people who are actively involved in their own spiritual journey. As one guide on spirituality and counseling notes:

> Counselors should be actively engaged in their own spiritual journey, one that includes practices congruent with the counselor's chosen spiritual path. In helping a client along his or her spiritual journey there is no substitute for personal experience.[8]

There is no demand that the clinician be 'religious' or even that they participate in a well-defined spiritual system. The clinician simply needs to be a person who is aware of the spiritual aspect of his or her personhood, and is actively seeking to nurture that part of the self. It would be very difficult for a person who denied the spiritual facet of the person, or avoided or repressed that aspect of the self, to work with others around spiritual issues.

Categories of interventions

It is possible to categorize interventions in many different ways. The preferred approach is to use the objective of the intervention to determine the category. The objectives, which we defined in Chapter 8, provide an excellent framework as they are progressive in nature and pull us toward our ultimate goal of healing. Early in the process, for example, we are trying to create awareness. Therefore we want to develop strategies that produce this desired result. Later, we might want to the patient to think about the beliefs and values they have disclosed. For this activity we need a different category of interventions: those that challenge the status quo and encourage critical reflection. Using this approach we can define the following categories.

Empathic strategies – creating trust
Gathering information/assessing – creating awareness
Challenging/reflecting – stimulating change
Facilitating spiritual movement – facilitating change
Collaborative strategies – facilitating change

As we develop strategies appropriate for each of these categories or stages, it is critical that we be aware of several other factors. These additional factors help us expand our thinking and become more creative and inclusive in our approaches.

First, as we choose to work with patients on spiritual issues we are not ultimately limited by the clinical setting or by our training and experience. It is possible to supplement what happens in a session with interventions that take place outside of the clinical setting. We can provide our patients with 'homework' or 'soul work,' prescribing activities they can do between clinical sessions. Those activities might include specific religious activities, such as worship, prayer, the reading of sacred writings from the person's faith system, or participation in sacraments or rituals. They might include more universal or esoteric exercises such as meditation, walking meditation, or reading from writings that are not aligned with a specific religion.

We can also augment our efforts by referring patients to spiritual resources that can aid them in their efforts to become whole. Those resources can be in the form of spiritual specialists, such as a religious leader or spiritual counselor, or they can be in the form of groups, such as 12-step groups, support groups, or study groups. Using such resources greatly enhances the limited training and experience of the healthcare professional. Such collaboration is critically important for the integration of spirituality and medicine, for without collaboration, the ability to impact patients spiritually is severely limited.

The use of spiritual interventions

We have already discussed the various levels of counseling, ranging from listening to psychotherapy. The interventions that are possible within the healthcare context will involve all three levels. The first two levels, active listening and providing counsel, are likely to take place in the healthcare setting itself and be implemented by the clinicians themselves. The third level, psychotherapy or formal spiritual counseling, is more likely to take place outside the clinical setting and be provided by spiritual experts or mental health professionals. These interventions will be the result of a referral by the healthcare professional, and, ideally, will be collaborative in nature.

Interventions to create trust

The first prerequisite of the effective integration of medicine and spirituality is the development of a safe environment. So many patients have no one they really trust. Such people have no relationship that provides them with a sense of security and comfort. The therapeutic relationship can become such a relationship. The physician, nurse, or social worker can help a patient feel cared for, valued, and safe. They can provide a context where the patient feels free to share his or her deepest thoughts and feelings. Thus, initial interventions must focus on creating that 'free and friendly space' where spiritual healing can occur.

The most basic of these interventions is what we have called *active listening* (Chapter 7). Listening is an act of love. By truly allowing the patient to say what they need and desire to say, but using techniques that allow them to maintain control of the conversation's agenda, we show that we care and that we value the thoughts feelings and perceptions of the other.

Empathy is also conveyed by the messages we send. It is conveyed first through body language: through eye contact, touch, by simply leaning forward. It is conveyed when we share, directly and clearly, our own internal state. When we have empathy our feelings mirror those of the person we listen to. What they are feeling at a deep level grabs us, and creates a similar feeling in us. This is why it is important, as one professor at a Princeton Seminary once said, to 'trust your tummies.'

> Neil was a first-year Family Medicine resident. He was in the middle of an obstetrical rotation when he was present at a spontaneous abortion. Plans were being made by the medical staff to autopsy the child and then dispose of the body. While talking to the mother he began to get a sense of deep anguish. He said to the young mother, who was numbly agreeing to the instructions of the surgeon in charge of the case, 'As I listen to you I feel a sense of real anguish. Is this how you feel too?' At this the young woman broke down. It turned out that in her faith system it was deemed very important for even a fetus to be given a 'Christian' service and be buried with the family. This related to the group's beliefs about resurrection of the body. It was very important to her to take her baby home, a need the obstetrical staff was ignoring.

Because Neil was able to experience genuine empathy, and was able to express that empathy through a direct expression of feeling, he was able to help a young woman share a critical spiritual issue.

With empathy we take what Lewis Walker calls the 'second position.' When we take this position, we imagine that we are in the other person shoes, 'feeling their feelings and thinking their thoughts.'[9] Walker suggests we use *I–You* statements to present the thoughts and feelings that arise when we take this unique perspective. We say in effect, '*I* sense how it has been for *You*.' It is important to note that when we share what we believe is their perspective, that we must do so in a tentative manner. As has been noted before, we cannot truly know their perspective. We can only guess. But it is appropriate to guess, as long as it involves an authentic effort to feel with the other person, and as long as we 'check' that perception. It is important then that any *I–You* statement include a check to make sure we have been reasonably accurate.

Empathy is the starting point for any spiritual intervention. It should also be the ending point. That is why the BATHE technique (Chapter 6) ends with an E for empathy. Once people have been open and have disclosed critical issues and feelings, it is important that they be assured that they have not only been heard, but heard with respect and compassion.

Interventions to gather information and create awareness

The act of gathering information is a necessary precursor to intervention, but such activities are also truly interventions in themselves. Many people have significant gaps in their self-awareness that involve powerful issues and feelings. The process of listening to others, and thinking critically about what they say, is one way to help them fill in those gaps: to bring what was hidden within to the surface, where it can be dealt with.

The process of gathering information involves, again, active listening. By using skills such as paraphrasing, perception checks, creative questions, and negative inquiry, we not only come to understand the patient, but we help that patient come to self-understanding. It is not unusual for a patient, who has been helped by the use of good listening skills to share more deeply, to suddenly arrive at self-understanding.

Bob came into his clinic suffering from severe neck pain. He was sure he had simply strained a muscle, and was looking for a muscle relaxant. As he and his physician discussed what was going on in this life, Bob's body language was extremely suggestive. He talked loudly and quickly, his face was tense, and he often clenched his fists. In addition, he made numerous negative remarks about his job. The physician, wanting to explore all possible factors contributing to Bob's condition, asked him if there were any stressors in his life.

Bob quickly answered in the negative. 'No! Things are fine.'

'I was just wondering,' the physician replied 'I couldn't help but notice that your voice has been rather loud, and you have been clenching your fists. [Behavior description] When I act that way it usually means I'm angry.'

Before the physician could even check his observations, Bob responded: 'Wow, I hadn't really thought about it, but you are right. I am really angry. I worked incredibly hard to get a project going at work. I go on a business trip for a couple days, and I find they've changed the project. Then I go to a planning meeting and find they cancelled the meeting, and didn't even bother to tell me. I can't believe they did that!'

Eventually the physician and Bob came to the conclusion that his neck pain had its genesis in the stress he was feeling at work. He was feeling threatened, vulnerable, unappreciated, and, above all, angry. Once he was able to identify his feelings he was able to respond to them in an effective manner. A spiritual person, he chose to see the situation as an opportunity to reassess his life and look for new directions. An outstanding program developer, he moved from his job with a large corporation and began work for a newly formed non-profit. His neck pain went away.

The process of gathering information and enabling awareness can also involve a number of strategies that are not contained within the clinical setting. As part of the process patients can be given 'homework': exercises or tasks which they do on their own. The results of these activities then become the focus of a later clinical session. One such tool is the development of spectrums such as those described in Chapter 7. The process is relatively simple. The patient is asked to think about their spiritual life and identify five to eight themes that they believe are important. These themes can be either positive or negative. Negative qualities are to be written on the left side of a piece of paper, and positive on the right. They are then to find a word that describes the opposite end of the spectrum, and write that one on the other side of the paper from the original word. The result is a set of polarities or spectrums. When these polarities are brought back at the next visit the patient has the opportunity to place themselves on each spectrum. This is a variant use of the spiritual spectrum discussed previously and has outstanding possibilities. The following is a set of spectrums, complete with commentary, that was brought in by one patient.

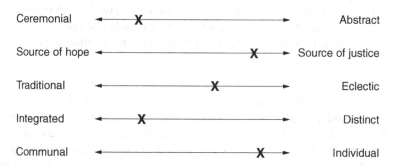

Figure 9.1

This particular patient not only created the spectrums, but added the following commentary to explain her choices.

- **Ceremonial/abstract:** The degree to which the person's spirituality is expressed in rituals.
- **Source of hope/source of justice:** The degree to which a person's spirituality offers hope or unwavering justice. A person whose spirituality is centered on hope, meaningfulness, and forgiveness is likely to construe their illness and its prognosis in a very different light than will a person whose spirituality is based in absolute justice and direct cause and effect.
- **Traditional/eclectic:** If a person's spiritual practices are conservative, it may be quite important to locate a spiritual adviser of their specific denomination/sect/ etc. However, a person with a more eclectic philosophy may be able to benefit from an ecumenical spiritual adviser or an adviser from a tradition different from their own.
- **Integrated/distinct:** These are my awkward terms for assessing the degree to which a person's spiritual values affect their daily life. Some people participate in a religious community as a social activity and do not consciously include spiritual considerations in their day-to-day decision making, while others see even the most minor decisions as having spiritual implications.
- **Communal/individual:** The degree to which a person is part of a community that shares their spiritual values. The community may be formally structured (for example, if the patient is a member of the Catholic Church) or loosely structured (the spiritual practices of many Native American people are like this).

While this particular person approached the task using a very objective, almost intellectual approach, the categories chosen were revealing and provided a great deal of understanding about this person's spirituality, which was based in the Native American culture.

Another tool that is often used to elicit awareness is journaling. The assignment is to write down any thoughts and feelings that occur, especially those related to spirituality, right at the moment of the thought. These thoughts are to be placed in context, with the surrounding circumstances also noted. The journal entries can be quickly reviewed and used as a starting point for discussion. The entries can be either positive or negative. Positive entries are important for they provide an understanding of the ways in which a person's spirituality is supporting them, and enabling them to cope with life. Negative entries are the equivalent of what might be called confession, a revealing of the dark, the failures, and the unpleasant. By acknowledging these things, gaining self-awareness, the door is opened to healing. To the extent that a failure, doubt, or negative feeling is known and examined, it may be changed or healed.

Another potential intervention would be to have patients develop a cognitive map of their spiritual journeys (this tactic can be used with both individuals and groups). This is the same exercise clinicians sometimes use to explore their own spirituality. The basic assignment is for the patient to record their spiritual journey, from their first awareness to the present moment. What were some of the key moments along the way? What impact did these key moments have? How did they affect the journey? The educational goal is to help the learners understand where they are at the current moment, as well as the process involved. What do they affirm, and why? What do they reject, find abhorrent, and why?

The goal of these interventions is to create awareness in both the clinician and the patient. What does the patient believe? What are his or her values? What are the basic underlying 'rules' that influence his life, for good or for ill? Through these interventions, the clinician begins to gain an understanding of the pivotal issues and, more importantly, the patient gains critical self-awareness. This awareness is a basic building block for transformation. As the knowledge is explored and the rules, beliefs, and values evaluated, the way is opened for change and growth.

Questions for reflection

- Have you ever had a moment when you suddenly became aware of a new truth about yourself, or aware of a feeling that had previously gone unnoticed?
- What was the catalyst that led to that new awareness?
- In what ways did that new awareness influence your current feelings, thoughts, or behaviors?

Interventions to stimulate reflection and change

The next set of interventions is designed to be evaluative in nature. These interventions involve a significant shift in characteristic as they are more proactive. The interventions related to information gathering intentionally leave the control of the encounter in the hands of the patient. These interventions, while respectful of the patient and non-coercive, are more directive. The free information offered by the patient is responded to in such a way as to amplify, challenge, and reframe.

Questioning focuses on the filtering patterns of deletion, generalization, and distortion. We have already proposed that it is important to notice when people omit information, fall into vague generalizations, or distort reality to fit their beliefs or values. Questioning not only notes the filtering pattern, but essentially challenges it.

For example, a person, when talking about God, might say, 'My relationship with God is not working.' This is a deletion because no insight is given into the nature of the relationship, or the nature of the problem. For clarification, we must know more. The appropriate intervention involves asking questions that fill in the gaps. 'In what ways is the relationship not satisfying?' 'What has happened that makes you feel your relationship with God is not healthy?'

The same basic strategy works when a patient generalizes. A patient says, 'I never do anything right?' This of course is an obvious example of a generalization. An effective intervention would clearly challenge this statement. It could be as simple as replying with 'Never?' Another patient might say, 'I just can't seem to be spiritual.' This generalization can be challenged simply by asking, 'What stops you?' The goal is both to gather more information and to break the patterns of thought that are limiting the patient from growth and healing.

Distortion, as we have noted, is when people change the meaning of an event to fit their own versions of reality. Most people don't recognize that their distortion is not, in fact, reality but merely their perception. Sometimes distortions take the form of mind reading. 'You hate me.' Or the patient may distort cause and effect, invalidly attaching either a cause to an effect or an effect to a cause by stating, 'I made God reject me.' When faced with what seems to be a distortion we can again ask clarifying questions. 'How do you know I hate you?' 'How exactly did you make God reject you?' Again the purpose of questioning the statement is to gain more information, challenge existing patterns of thought, and open up new options.

Ready and Burton, in their book on neuro-linguistic programming, offer the following suggestions to those who would deal with universal patterns, or what they call 'the Meta Model.' First, if multiple patterns are present, they suggest clinicians 'challenge distortions first, then generalizations, and then deletions.' If one starts with deletions, they caution, he or she may get more information than can be processed. The process as they define it is simple – first listen actively and spot the pattern, then intervene with the right question(s).[10]

A similar tactic involves directly challenging irrational ideas and moving the patient toward more rational, less self-defeating ideas. In his book *Reason and Emotion in Psychotherapy*, Albert Ellis identifies a number of what he calls irrational ideas. That list includes the following.

1 It is a dire necessity for me to be loved or approved of by everyone for everything I do.
2 It is easier to avoid than to face life difficulties and self-responsibilities.
3 I should be thoroughly competent, adequate, intelligent, and successful in all possible respects.
4 Human happiness can be achieved by inertia and inaction.
5 Because something once strongly affected my life, it should indefinitely affect it.

It is clear how such thoughts could well create significant problems. No person, for example, can live up to the standard of being loved or approved of by everyone for everything her or she does. Trying to live up to that 'life rule' will create frustration and probably lead to hopelessness. Similar problematic ideas can emerge from the spiritual realm. 'God demands righteousness, any time a person is not righteous, God punishes.' We hesitate to call them irrational, since what is irrational to one faith system may seem perfectly logical to another. But we can certainly classify them as problematic if they involve standards or ideas that are inherently defeating. The key is the impact the belief or value has on the patient. If it is causing dis-ease, if it is hindering their ability to feel connected to the sacred or other, or if it causes them to be 'stuck,' unable to move forward to healing, then it is a problematic thought.

When such an idea is expressed, the clinician's goal is to help the patient rethink the rule. One effective way to intervene when faced with problematic thoughts is to use what one author calls the A-B-C-D-E system:[11]

- A stands for activating event
- B stands for belief system
- C stands for consequences
- D stands for disputing the problematic idea
- E stands for new emotional consequence or effect.

The following dialogue illustrates how this system might be used in the clinical setting.

> **Patient:** I should have known I would get something like cancer. I knew God would eventually punish me for failing to be righteous.
> **Clinician:** Well, you seem to believe that your cancer is somehow connected to your behavior, and that God has caused it. Are you actually saying that this cancer is your fault?
> **Patient:** Well, I know God is angry with me, and I've always believed that something like this would happen.
> **Clinician:** It seems like you are struggling with the news you have received, and that you are trying to find a reason for the cancer afflicting you. It also seems that you have regrets about the way you have lived and believe God is angry at you. Let's think about these ideas for a moment. Let's start with the event (A) that started this chain of thoughts, that's your bone cancer. To that you've added the belief (B) that God wants to punish you for the way you've lived. This has resulted in you thinking (C) that the cancer is God's punishment of an unloved person. Let's think about those beliefs again. What makes you think you've deserved God's anger and that the cancer comes from God?
> **Patient:** I'm not totally sure. But I look at the Bible and I look at other Christians and I know my life just doesn't measure up. So I just put two and two together...
> **Clinician:** I'm sorry, but I just can't agree with you. I understand your feeling that you may not have lived an exemplary life. But I just can't make the connection between that and your cancer. Your type of cancer happens to all kinds of people. I wonder if instead of telling yourself your cancer is a sign God is angry, you can tell yourself the cancer is just a bad event, and that God, rather than being angry, is sorrowful, and wants to be with you and for you? (D) And I'm wondering in what ways

you feel your life is not good enough. Is it possible your expectations are too high?

Hopefully such a discussion, which is brief and entirely possible within a clinical session, would begin to effect (E) a new emotional state for the client, that of hope rather than despair.

Another intervention that can be used within a clinical session is that of 'reframing.' As one source defines it, '"reframing" is a psychotherapeutic intervention which can address complex relationship dynamics, especially at times when it appears that coping and adjustment are being thwarted by reliance on unhelpful beliefs. Reframing as an intervention serves to introduce new views and possibilities.'[12] The key to reframing is helping people understand they can deal with issues when they have a balanced view of that issue. It is when a person is trapped on one end of a spectrum that they lose options. As Propst notes, 'Dysfunction, distortion, and pain result when our thinking in any of these categories is at one of the polar extremes.'[13] Death, for example, can best be explored in the context of Life. A sense of being alone or disconnected can be comprehended more fully in the context of connectedness.

When people have unhelpful beliefs about their problems, one task of the healer is to offer alternative views when suitable. This is done by addressing both sides of a particular theme. The objective is to reframe one side of the problem in the context of the other. As Bor *et al.* suggest:

> Discussing the complementary aspects of an idea can help to change the patient's perceptions of a problem, leading to emotional and behavioural change. This can be achieved where the patient comes to a different understanding of his situation by making new connections and recognizing alternative but plausible perspectives to a problem. In the seemingly hopeless situation of a fatal illness, a patient may, for example, recognize the extent of caring and closeness in his family for the first time.[14]

With this process the clinician does not invalidate the existing perspective held by the patient, but 'balances' that perspective with the appropriate complement. This helps to move the person to what might be called 'middle ground.' The patient's view of the problem must not be invalidated. The end of the spectrum the patient has embraced should not be denied or rejected. Instead the patient's perspective is to be expanded, carefully and with great sensitivity, to include more than the original polar extreme.

This approach is extremely helpful when a person's condition is life changing (permanent), chronic, or terminal. For people whose disease has them focused on death or dying, helping to balance their views and begin to think once again about life and living can be enabling.

Patient: So, I'm going to die, there is nothing you can do?
Clinician: From all the tests, I believe that this syndrome will eventually lead to your death. But there are always things we can do to help. We might be able to slow the progress of the disease down. We can work to preserve your function and we can control many of the symptoms. I think, realistically, you have between six months and a year, based upon your current condition.

Patient: Well I guess that's it.

Clinician: How are you feeling right now?

Patient: Numb. A bit frightened

Clinician: What is it that frightens you?

Patient: Death. No, not exactly the actual fact of dying, but the process of dying. My situation is hopeless. There is nothing I can do. What will my pitiful future be like? All I can see at this point is the fact that I will, month by month, slowly become less functional. Pretty soon I'll just be a lump of flesh.

Clinician: It is frightening to think about the progression of such a disease. I can certainly understand your fear. But I am wondering – are there ways in which you can see yourself taking advantage of the time you have left? Are there things you'd like to do?

Patient: Well, it is hard to get past what I am losing. I really love walking, getting outside in nature, but I just can't do that anymore, I always fall.

Clinician: I know it is hard to walk right now. But I think we should find ways to help you keep living, and do the things that are important to you. Let's look at some options…

It would be foolish to suggest that by helping patients find balance we will magically solve their problems. This process may well be merely an initial step toward wholeness, and it may take ongoing effort and specialized help for the process to be completed. Still, the process has the potential to create a new openness and receptivity to options.

Those interventions focused on facilitating active reflection about beliefs and values are certainly not inclusive. But these strategies are brief and are not overly complex. More sophisticated tools belong to the realm of psychotherapy and are not generally appropriate for the integration of spirituality into the healthcare setting.

Questions for reflection

- Think of a person who clearly used one of the universal filters (distortion, deletion, or generalization). What would an effective challenge/question be for that statement?
- Think of an 'unhelpful' thought or life rule that you have heard a patient express. Why do you think the rule is 'unhelpful?' Use the A-B-C-D-E tool to craft a response to that statement that would help the patient to a new stance.
- Think of a key issue that you think influences your patients (or yourself). What is the complement of that issue? (For example, the complement for hopeless is hopeful.) Imagine your self being out of balance. What does it feel like to live on one end of the spectrum? What would it mean to move into a balanced position? How would that impact your potential options?

Interventions to stimulate change and growth

It usually is not the role of healthcare professionals to provide long-term therapy. They have neither the time nor the training needed for intense and complicated spiritual counseling. This does not mean, however, that they cannot be catalysts for change. Already, by helping to create awareness and by questioning and challenging the beliefs and values of their patients, they have initiated the process of healing. Awareness alone may be all that is needed Once aware of the issues at hand, the patients can move forward to create solutions for themselves. At other times, the patient may need additional input, such as disputing and questioning, to move toward spiritual healing. And, in some cases, it may be necessary and helpful to introduce interventions that have a healing focus. Some of these interventions may be focused on the clinical session, while others may involve homework or referral. The common denominator is that these interventions tend to involve actions that are beneficial to people from a spiritual and, at times, physical perspective.

One such intervention involves what are commonly called **relaxation techniques**. Perhaps the most well-known proponent of this intervention is Herbert Benson MD, of Harvard Medical School. Benson is convinced that a person benefits greatly when they integrate spirituality into the healing process. As he reflects upon his own professional development he notes the following:

> I became convinced that our bodies are wired to benefit from exercising not only our muscles but our rich inner, human core – our beliefs, values, thoughts, and feelings ... I could not shake the sense I had the human mind – and the beliefs we so often associate with the human soul – had physical manifestations.[15]

One of the interventions Benson believes is most effective is relaxation techniques. These techniques facilitate what he labels the 'relaxation response.' According to Benson 'the human body is geared to react by providing this calming state ... whenever the mind is focused for some time and disregards intrusive, everyday thoughts. In other words, when the mind quiets down the body follows suit.'[16]

There are a number of procedures for facilitating relaxation that can be used within the context of spirituality. One such procedure is very physical in nature. The patient is asked to tighten a muscle, focusing on the tension. Then the tension is slowly released and the focus of attention moves to the sensation of relaxation, with an awareness of the differences between the states of tension and relaxation. This total body exercise can be taught quickly in the clinical setting, and then used by the patient at home. Later, the patient is asked to tighten and relax muscles in sequence, starting with the hands, moving up the arms to the face, then moving down to the chest, abdomen, and finally the legs and feet.

Jim Gordon, in his Mind/Body seminars,[17] teaches a technique that involves relaxation only. The patient is taught a sequence of phrases which they repeat to themselves for the purpose of relaxing the body and dilating the veins. The process follows a sequence similar to that used above and goes as follows.[18]

1 Take a few minutes to concentrate on relaxing your whole body. Shake your shoulders, inhale and exhale deeply and slowly a few times, and clear your mind of thoughts and concerns.

2   Next, focus your attention on your left arm and repeat to yourself over and over that it is getting heavy and it is getting warm. Continue this repetition until you actually feel that your left arm has become very heavy and very warm.

3   Do this for your right arm, each of your legs, your stomach, your chest, your neck, your head, and your face. Focus your attention on each body area in turn, repeating that it is getting very heavy and very warm.

4   Continue this relaxation until you feel the tension flow out of you. Feel the tension flow into the couch or the bed you are lying on. (You may fall asleep during all this, but it's more likely you'll feel awake, but very quiet in body and mind.) Let yourself rest there, quiet and relaxed, for 10 minutes or so. You will feel calm and refreshed when you arise. (Note: this relaxation technique gets easier and more beneficial each time you use it.)

Often this technique is used with a surface thermometer to provide the patient with tangible evidence of its impact on the body. Such techniques have many characteristics of self-hypnosis and often mirror commonly used techniques of trance induction.

Another potential intervention involves the use of **spiritual exercises**. These exercises can be 'denominational' or 'ecumenical.' Denominational exercises may involve activities or rituals related to a specific religious perspective. Ecumenical exercises will be broader and have a universal application. This is a very useful approach for people who are depressed or feeling frozen spiritually. By picking tasks that help patients gain knowledge or information and nurture the spiritual side of their beings, we can help them move forward and successfully implement a new option. The process is relatively simple. The first step is to work with the patient to define a problem that needs to be addressed, or a positive goal that the person would like to reach. The next step is to define a strategy to solve the problem or reach the goal, and divide that strategy into specific stages. The development of these stages is very important. For more complex projects, a larger number of stages should be developed. The condition of the patient will also affect the number of stages, and thus the rate of change. An individual who is very vulnerable or shy might need to take smaller steps. A small step, successfully accomplished, is better than a larger step that is unreachable.

One woman felt that she was incapable of building meaningful relationships. She felt she could not develop friendships, but extended that sense of incompetence to doubting her intimate relationships and her relationship to the sacred. As a result she felt very disconnected, and visited her family medicine clinic with vague complaints. Her family physician had become a primary connection in her life. Once her sense of isolation was understood, her family physician helped her set an initial goal of meeting more people and establishing one new friendship. The first small step was merely to gather the telephone number of some singles' groups in her community. Given her spiritual history, the step was even more defined, as only faith-based groups were to be included in the initial effort.

Once the goals and action steps have been developed, then it is helpful to identify rewards for the completion of each step. Since people struggling with dis-ease may have difficulty giving themselves positive rewards, this can be an added thera-peutic element. The rewards should be chosen by the patient. In the case above, the first award was a new dress.

The simple task of connecting to another person would be a beginning step. A next step might involve using a spiritual exercise out of that person's faith perspective as a way of building a relationship with the divine. One physician used the simple tactic of having a patient read the Old Testament psalms. One psalm was read at the beginning of each week, with the patient looking at both the nature of the psalmist (who in most cases is far from perfect) and the response of God (which is graceful and restorative). Indeed, encouraging patients to read books that address their spiritual issues is a solid way to create growth and movement, provided the books are compatible with the patient's spiritual background.

Meditation is a widely acclaimed intervention that crosses many spiritual per-spectives and can have a variety of forms and purposes. It can be used for relaxation, awareness, and centering. It can be used to focus on God. In mind/body medicine it is used to facilitate healing in the body.[19] Most definitions of meditation address the concept that meditation helps a person focus their attention. Some definitions include the following.

- Meditation is focusing one's attention in one direction.[20]
- Meditation is 'consciously directing your attention to alter your state of con-sciousness.'[21]
- Meditation is 'Sitting still, doing nothing.'[22]
- Meditation focuses on 'quieting the busy mind.'[23]

Meditation can be implemented in a variety of settings. Some clinicians will lead their patients through a meditation within a clinical session. Others will provide a taped meditation experience for the patient to use, either in the clinic or at home. Others will teach patients meditative techniques and encourage them to use those techniques regularly between clinical sessions. It is also possible to use meditation in a group setting.

Many websites provide training in meditative techniques, as well as specific meditations. Training in meditative techniques specifically focused on physical and mental health clinicians is available through organizations such as Jim Gordon's Center for Mind-Body Medicine[24] and Herbert Benson's Mind/Body Medical Institute.[25] In some communities meditation groups are available through local organizations, including religious groups, non-profits, and even health systems.

It is a fallacy to believe that interventions using meditation are complex or difficult. Herbert Benson often uses a simple meditation process that takes no more than 15 to 20 minutes.[26] Only a quiet environment is needed: a setting where one can be quiet, undisturbed, and in a comfortable position. The process has two simple steps: the silent repetition of a word, sound, phrase, or prayer; and the passive return to the repetition whenever other thoughts intrude. The simplicity of these instructions makes this technique available to virtually anyone, regardless of spiritual or religious beliefs. This is because the person can use as their repetitive focus a prayer or any other words that reinforce their beliefs (e.g. 'God is love').

Mindfulness meditation is another popular approach to meditation that involves the ability to focus completely on only one thing at a time. In other words, the mind is full of whatever is happening right now. This can include walking, cooking, sweeping the floor, dancing, watching a bird, hearing the sound of a river, or any other focus a person chooses. Whenever stray thoughts intrude, the person simply returns his or her focus to the current moment. This is a traditional Buddhist approach, and has been widely popularized by Jon Kabat-Zinn PhD in the Stress Reduction Clinic at the University of Massachusetts Medical Center in Worcester.[27]

With guided meditation, a leader or tape provides the patient with a sequence of instructions that shape the content of the experience. The following meditation is one suggested by the Center for Mind-Body Medicine. It is used during their training seminars and is posted on their website.[28]

Allow yourself to sit back and relax – Loosen any clothing that feels tight – remove your glasses if you wish – see that your arms and your legs are in a position that feels right for you. And if you are comfortable with it, slowly and gently close your eyes.

And allow your attention to move to your breathing. Let your breathing become even and comfortable. Breathing is one of the most powerful conscious influences you have on your nervous system.

So now I'd like you to see yourself in a very special place ... it could be a real place – a place you may actually have been – a beautiful spot in nature or comforting place in your own home. Your special place may be an imaginary place – a place in fairy tales – indoors or outdoors – it doesn't really matter. Should more than one place come to mind, allow yourself to stay with one of them.

The only thing that matters is that it is a place in which you are completely comfortable and safe... You feel comfortable and safe. Appreciate this scene with all of your senses. Hear the sounds – smell the aromas, feel the air as it caresses your skin – experience the ground securely under you – touch and feel the whole environment that you are in.

Notice what you are wearing.

Notice what you have on your feet.

What time of year it is, what time of day.

How old you are.

Whether you are alone or with another person or people.

Notice the colors that surround you.

What is the temperature? Is it warm? Is it cold?

Notice the qualities of the place that make it safe and comfortable.

And look around you to see if there is anything else that would make this place more safe for you... Perhaps something that you need to remove from the place or something you need to bring in... And then notice how your body feels in this place... and now take some time to enjoy this feeling of safety in your special place...

And now thank yourself for taking the time ... this time for yourself ... and perhaps promising yourself, and reassuring yourself that you will visit this place or some other place on your own, whenever you need to.

And when you're ready ... at your own pace ... let your breathing deepen... Very gradually let the awareness of your body against the chair return... Bring yourself back slowly and comfortably... And now when you are ready ... and only when you are ready ... gently open your eyes with a smile on your face.

Guided imagery can have very specific spiritual content if it is deemed appropriate. For example, one physician, when working with Christian clients, guides them down a road where they meet and talk with the resurrected Christ. Another has patients go to a 'special place' and in the unique environment meet and talk with a 'special person,' a spiritual mentor, God, Jesus, Buddha, whomever they want to place in that role.

Many of those involved in the mind-body medicine movement make wide use of mental imagery as a type of meditative technique. Mental imagery involves using mental pictures to imagine changes in the body. Sometimes the person simply does a body scan. Starting in the head, they imagine themselves being able to move down through the body, seeing the bones, muscles, and organs, imagining the entire body as healthy and whole. If there is an illness, they are asked to focus on that illness. A person, for example, with a tumor, can imagine that tumor, aided by a description provided by the physician, and then picture that tumor shrinking, disappearing. A patient with chronic pain might imagine that pain is melting away and dripping like a warm liquid out of their body. This is a highly personalized technique, and the patient would use images that are uniquely exciting and meaningful to them. Again, many of the principles of clinical hypnosis are integrated into this approach.

Studies of mental imagery have found that people can actually influence their immune functioning as well as significantly reduce pain and tension in the body with this method.[29] But aside from the physiological benefits, which take some practice to achieve, there is also the benefit of the person feeling empowered, having that sense that they have been able to channel their energy into a healing activity.

Certainly, when talking about spirituality and healing, we would be remiss if we did not mention **prayer**. Many faith traditions, and many people, consider prayer an important resource with respect to healing. According to Gallup, 90% of Americans pray. Of those who pray, 97% believe their prayers are heard and 95% believe they are answered.[30] When a group of seriously ill pulmonary patients were surveyed, 90% said they believe prayer could aid in recovery.[31] When a group of hospitalized patients were asked about effective pain management strategies, 64% said prayer was a critical management mechanism. It was third, topped only by pain pills (82%) and IV pain mediation (66%).[32]

Prayer is for many, patients and clinicians alike, an effective intervention. Some clinicians, if requested, find it meaningful to pray with their patients. This prayer can be spoken, or it can be a matter of prayerful silence. In some cases, clinicians who are not comfortable praying with a patient will offer that patient the freedom to pray, and then will sit with the patient in empathic silence. Others refer the patient to a chaplain if one is available.

We must be careful with this particular intervention. A recent article on professional boundaries notes that 'a physician who initiates prayer without first being asked presents an ethical problem because patients might easily feel coerced.'[33] The authors of this study eventually concluded that in most cases it is best for the physician not to pray with their patients.

> Physician-led prayer is acceptable only when pastoral care is not readily available, when the patient is intent on prayer with the physicians, and when the physician can pray without having to feign faith and without manipulating the patient. Under these circumstances, one recommendation

that is acceptable to the secular physician is to simply listen respectfully as a patient prays.[34]

In the hospital, it is most appropriate to refer those who desire prayer to the chaplains. The physician may choose to stay with the family and patient while the chaplain offers the prayer. In the cases where there is no other option, physician–patient prayer must be done with authenticity or not at all.

Many clinicians find the most appropriate use of this intervention is to pray *for* their patients, within the context of their own spiritual perspective, rather than to pray *with* them. The key to this intervention is to make sure it is patient-centered (and is about their faith not ours) and is respectful of each person's belief system.

Certainly the suggestions offered here regarding healing interventions are only representative of the possible options. It is our hope that these ideas provide a starting place to develop your own set of interventions. Remember that each person is different. Interventions should be chosen carefully to be respectful of the person's unique spiritual culture. Always check with the patient about their interest in such an intervention. In the context of a relationship built on trust, it is possible to have an honest discussion with patients about the degree to which they would like spirituality integrated into their care. It is noteworthy that both of the mnemonics (HOPE and FICA) provided earlier in the book end with a question about whether the patient would like to address spirituality as part of their treatment.

Collaborative interventions

As we have noted before, the degree to which clinicians can address spirituality in the healthcare setting is limited by such factors as training, time, and the acceptance of their health system. Even if they choose to address spiritual issues as part of the therapeutic process, there comes a point when the needs go beyond the capacity of the physician to meet them.

Just as there are times when a clinician must refer to a specialist because of the complexity of the physical condition, so there are times when the clinician must refer to a specialty because of the spiritual condition. When this time comes there are actually many options.

If the patient is in a hospital or nursing home, a **chaplain** may be available. Chaplains are spiritual specialists trained to address spiritual needs in the healthcare setting. They are highly trained and, as part of their code of ethics, committed to affirming 'the religious and spiritual freedom of all persons.' They also pledge that they will refrain from imposing doctrinal positions or spiritual practices on persons whom they encounter in their professional role as chaplain.[35] This inherent respect for the spiritual culture of the patient makes a chaplain an excellent resource. Clinicians with hospitalized patients can refer patients with spiritual issues to the chaplain program confident that the approach will be appropriate. As with any referral, it is important to get the patient's permission to make that referral. Chaplains also make the rounds of the various wards and offer patients their services in a direct manner. In some cases chaplains will discuss a critical issue with a patient and, with the patient's permission, inform the physician of that issue as it relates to recovery. We strongly suggest that clinicians become familiar with the chaplain services at the hospitals to which they admit patients. The development of a professional relationship with the chaplains will aid in both consultation and collaboration.

Another critical resource may well be **local religious leaders**. They provide services to patients being referred from outpatient settings and to patients in smaller communities where there are no professional chaplains. It is important to refer patients only to those leaders who are appropriate for the patient's unique spiritual culture. If a person has a pastor, rabbi, or other such leader, they will probably be the best referral option. There may be instances when this is not the case. If the spiritual issue has strong moral or ethical overtones, the patient may not want to deal with that issue within their own community of faith. One patient, dealing with a great deal of guilt over an extramarital affair and subsequent sexually transmitted disease, preferred to talk about that issue with someone other than his own pastor.

Again, it is important for healthcare professionals to become familiar with the religious leaders in their community. In small communities, it may be helpful to meet with most of the leaders personally. One physician, upon moving to a new community, invited each of the religious leaders, including all of the various Christian ministers and a Buddhist monk, to join him, one by one, for a short meeting. Over coffee or lunch they had the opportunity to talk about how they envisioned working together. Although one pastor stated quite clearly that he didn't want the physician to 'mess with' his parishioners, most of the encounters were very useful. This kind of tactic may not be practical in a larger community.

In general, it is good, even in larger communities, to find clergy who are open to and appreciative of the process of counseling and nurturing of those in their care. This process of referral to local clergy is not easy. There is the issue of confidentiality. If the patient is not part of a faith community, it may be difficult to ensure that the patient follows up with the spiritual leader's care. It may be difficult or impossible to get information back from the pastor. In spite of these difficulties collaborative care with a spiritual leader can be a critical and powerful intervention.

In some communities, there is a group of persons called '**spiritual counselors**.' This term can mean many different things. Sometimes a person called a spiritual counselor is really a minister on a church staff who does 'counseling.' This person may, or may not, have formal training in counseling techniques. If they are attached to a denomination, it may be best to limit referrals to those from that denomination. In other instances, spiritual counselors are licensed therapists or counselors who intentionally integrate ideas of spirituality in counseling. In other instances, spiritual counselors are people who focus on chakras, auras, energy medicine, healing touch, and other such 'spiritual' approaches. For some people, this kind of approach may be very appropriate, while for others it would be totally inappropriate. When making a referral it is important, again, to know something about the counselor involved so that you can make the appropriate referral based upon the patient's spiritual culture. One general quality we seek in any counselor is a willingness to be patient-centered. Spirituality means different things to different people. Therefore, it is important that the counselor first assess the client's beliefs to know how to proceed with the therapy.

Mind-body medicine focuses on the interactions among the brain, mind, body, and behavior, and the powerful ways in which emotional, mental, social, spiritual, and behavioral factors can directly affect health. It regards as fundamental an approach that respects and enhances each person's capacity for self-knowledge and self-care, and it emphasizes techniques that are grounded in this approach.

Mind-body practitioners can include physicians who add various mind-body techniques to their array of tools, social workers, psychotherapists, spiritual practitioners, and those who teach or lead practices such as yoga. There is currently no easy way to define local resources, other than taking the time to research those resources through the use of the internet and the phone book. However, finding mind-body practitioners can be exceptionally helpful for physicians who would like to provide mind-body interventions for their patients. Although many clinicians do learn to use these techniques themselves, some find it more helpful to find others who can provide this kind of care as a collaborator.

Referrals can be made to **groups** as well as to individual counselors or guides. Often there are a variety of groups available to those patients who need and want to do spiritual work. There are support groups and study groups. One church in Portland, Oregon has an ongoing group for people who have suffered a significant loss. The loss may be due to a death, but is not restricted to that scenario. People who have lost a relationship, for example, might also be involved in this group. The group is lay led and rarely has a planned agenda. It is a time for sharing and learning. People tell stories, sharing both struggles and successes. They read passages from sacred texts, or from other writings that have been helpful to them. They often engage in group meditation. Such a group might be a wonderful referral for a patient who is struggling with loss and grief. Again, the key is knowing what is available. One office in a moderate-sized community has the front office staff do research to discover all of the groups available in its community. The list is updated regularly. Each clinician is given a copy of the list, which provides the name of the group, its focus, and contact information.

When it comes to spirituality, the role of the healthcare clinician is, primarily, as a catalyst. Thus, the art of referral is one that should be nurtured. Little has been written about this important activity, and it appears that it is inconsistently carried out, especially in the outpatient setting. As we reflect upon this task, it appears a number of issues are dominant.

- First, it is important to know what resources are available in the community.
- Second, it is important to develop an appropriate method for referral. This method may need to be negotiated with the religious leaders and counselors themselves. How do they want to be contacted? What do they charge? What is the best way to ensure that the patient follows up on the referral? There are many details that need to be worked out.
- Third, it is critical to define how information will move back and forth between the healthcare professional and the spiritual specialist. What information will the healthcare provider give to the specialist? What kind of authorizations or permissions need to be in place? How will information be given back to the healthcare clinician? In other words, what kind of continuity and follow-up will be possible?

These issues must be addressed to move the integration of spirituality and medicine forward.

We recommend that any clinician who is thinking about the integration of healthcare and spirituality think in terms of a multidisciplinary care team. It is this team that provides the wide range of expertise and variety of settings that help people identify, address, and resolve spiritual, emotional, relational, and physical distress. Although a healer may do a great deal on his or her own, it is important not to narrow one's vision of what can occur to include only that which can be done alone. In terms of the integration of spirituality and healthcare, less is not more.

Summary

This book is all about the patient. We believe that it is important, first, to understand the patient as a whole person, not just as a physical entity with a disease. Patients must be seen as complex and multifaceted beings who must be treated in a holistic manner. All aspects of the self, the physical, social, emotional, and spiritual, are intrinsically related and impact one another. Thus, in the treatment of patients all these aspects must be explored and addressed. To treat patients from only the biomedical perspective is to turn them into a cadaver.

It is also important to remember that each person is unique. Each patient who walks through the door of a clinic for treatment has a unique personal culture. We must take care to understand that culture as we work with them. A part of that personal culture is an equally unique spiritual culture. Any attempt to work with a person around spiritual issues without first examining, to at least some degree, this culture is dangerous and inappropriate. And it is from the perspective of the patient's culture that all efforts must progress.

The goal is to help the patient move toward healing. Healing, we must remember, is sometimes distinct from cure. It involves finding such things as hope, love, and empowerment in the midst of illness, which is a state created by both physical disease and internal turmoil or dis-ease.

In order to move toward this goal we must accomplish three major tasks. First, we must gather information. We must work with the patient so that we both gain an understanding of what is happening physically and spiritually. In this process both the patient and the clinician gain a new level of awareness – in most cases both about themselves and the other. Second, we must think about our new knowledge. What is going on here? What is happening spiritually that either aids or hinders the healing process? What needs to be nurtured and supported and what needs to be challenged and changed? Third, there must be action. Clinicians and patients must affirm and encourage what is working. In other instances clinicians and patients must take action to facilitate change and growth. In many cases the therapeutic relationship expands at this point to include others, such as families, chaplains, spiritual leaders, and counselors.

This is important work. We approach it for many reasons. We seek this integration of spirituality into healthcare partly because it works and partly because patients find it meaningful – but mostly we do it because it adds a new dimension, a new depth to the process of healing. In a way it is, as James Gordon insists, 'a new medicine.'

> The new medicine that we are creating together appreciates the great value of surgery and drugs but sees them as last resorts, not first choices. It makes use of the most sophisticated modern diagnostic techniques and research studies, but also puts value on the learning and experience that humans in all parts of the world have accumulated over millennia.

> This new medicine understands that each of us ... is unique, a whole person – biological, psychological, spiritual – in a total social and ecological environment. It acknowledges that each of these dimensions of our lives can be both a source of our distress and an arena for relieving it... [36]

In a way, what we are talking about is also the 'old medicine.' It is a combining of the advances of modern sciences with the wisdom of the ages and the inner soul.

This is not about religious agendas. It is not about the beliefs and values of one person being imposed on another. It is about physicians and patients working together to find life and healing in the face of death and illness. It is about the 'art' of healing. William Blake in his poem 'Auguries of Innocence' writes:

> He who binds to himself a joy,
> Does the winged life destroy;
> But he who kisses the joy as it flies,
> Lives in eternity's sunrise.

It is our hope that this book will enable healers of all types to remember that newness and life, not permanence and death, are at the heart of what they do, and to find new depth and joy, and new satisfaction and effectiveness as they practice their art.

Notes

1 As quoted in Brown C (1998) *Afterward, You're a Genius*. Riverhead Books, New York, NY, p.292.

2 Christie RJ and Hoffmaster CB (1986) *Ethical Issues in Family Medicine*. Oxford University Press, New York, NY, pp.175–7.

3 Ellis M, Vinson D and Ewigman B (1999) Addressing spiritual concerns with patients: family physicians attitudes and practices. *J Fam Pract*. **48**(2): 105–9.

4 Levinson W, Gorawara-Bhat R and Lamb J (2000) A study of patient clues and physician responses in primary care and surgical settings. *JAMA*. **284**(8): 1021–7.

5 Koenig HG, McCullough ME and Larson DB (2001) *Handbook of Religion and Health*. Oxford University Press, New York, NY, pp.437–9.

6 Johnson AH (2001) The Balint Movement in America. *Fam Med*. **33**(3): 174–7.

7 Fukuyama MA and Sevig TD (1999) *Integrating Spirituality Into Multicultural Counseling*. Sage Publications, Thousand Oaks, CA.

8 Favier C, Ingersoll RE, O'Brien E and McNally C (2001) *Explorations in Counseling and Spirituality*. Brooks/Cole (Thomson Learning), Toronto, Canada, p.118.

9 Walker L (2002) *Consulting with NLP: neuro-linguistic programming in the medical consultation*. Radcliffe Medical Press, Oxford, p.120.

10 Ready R and Kate B (2004) *Neuro-linguistic Programming for Dummies*. John Wiley & Sons Ltd, Chichester, England, pp.234–5.

11 Okun BF (1997) *Effective Helping, Interviewing and Counseling Techniques* (5e). Brooks/Cole Publishing, Pacific Grove, CA, p.165.

12 Bor R, Miller R, Latz M and Salt H (1998) *Counseling in Health Care Settings*. Cassell, New York, NY, p.31.

13 Propst LR (1988) *Psychotherapy in a Religious Framework*. Human Sciences Press, New York, NY, p.100.

14 Bor R, Miller R, Latz M and Salt H (1998) *Counseling in Health Care Settings*. Cassell, New York, NY, p.32.

15 Benson H (1997) *Timeless Healing: the power and biology of belief*. Fireside Books (Simon & Schuster), New York, NY, p.17.

16 Benson H (1997) *Timeless Healing: the power and biology of belief*. Fireside Books (Simon & Schuster), New York, NY, p.127.

17 For information about Gordon's workshops for professionals, visit the Center for Mind-Body Medicine website at www.cmbm.org.

18 http://uasteph.tripod.com/Relaxation.htm. This exercise is from a site called 'Beyond the Body Betrayed.' The site was developed by a 21-year-old female who has struggled with a number of spiritual, mental, and emotional issues and is in recovery.

19 An excellent overview of the various kinds of meditation can be found at www.meditationcenter.com.

20 Propst LR (1988) *Psychotherapy in a Religious Framework*. Human Sciences Press, New York, NY, p.86.

21 www.meditationcenter.com.

22 A Taoist definition quoted on http://1stholistic.com/meditation.

23 Quoted on http://1stholistic.com/meditation. Another useful site is www.meditation society.com.

24 Information about the Center for Mind-Body Medicine can be found at www. cmbm.org. See also Gordon JS (1996) *Manifesto for a New Medicine*. Addison-Wesley Publishing Co, Reading, MA.

25 www/mbmi.org.

26 Benson H (1997) *Timeless Healing: the power and biology of belief*. Fireside Books (Simon & Schuster), New York, NY, Chapter 6.

27 Information about this center may be found at www.umassmededu/cfm/srp.

28 www.cmbm.org.

29 Zachariae R, Kristensen JS, Hockland P, Ellegaard J, Metze E and Hokland M (1990) Effect of psychological intervention in the form of relaxation and guided imagery on cellular immune function in normal healthy subjects. *Psychotherapy and Psychosomatics*. **54**: 32–9; also Auerbach JE, Oleson TD and Solomon GF (1992) A behavioral medicine intervention as an adjunctive treatment for HIV related illness. *Psychology and Health*. **6**: 325–34.

30 Gallup G Jr and Lindsay MD (1999) *Surveying the Religious Landscape*. Morehouse Publishing, Harrisburg, PA, p.45.

31 Ehman JW, Ott BB and Short TH (1999) Do patients want physicians to inquire about their spiritual or religious beliefs if they become gravely ill? *Arch Intern Med*. **159**(15): 1803–6.

32 McNeill JA *et al.* (1998) *Journal of Pain and Symptom Management*. **16**(1): 29–40.

33 Post SG, Puchalski CM and Larson DB (2000) Physicians and patient spirituality: professional boundaries, competency, and ethics. *Annals of Internal Medicine*. **132**(7): 578–83.

34 Post SG, Puchalski CM and Larson DB (2000) Physicians and patient spirituality: professional boundaries, competency, and ethics. *Annals of Internal Medicine*. **132**(7): 578–83.

35 From the Code of Ethics of the Association of Professional Chaplains.

36 Gordon JS (1996) *Manifesto for a New Medicine*. Addison-Wesley, Reading, MA, pp.17–18.

Epilogue

We hope that this book has helped to create a foundation for learning and talking about spirituality and medicine. In all likelihood, the reader had at least a passing interest in these issues before choosing to read this book. If so, you were probably halfway there before you even started to read. We have tried to outline an argument about why spirituality and medicine must work more closely together than we have in the past. As Americans live longer, and hopefully healthier, lives, the search for meaning in those lives will only intensify. Neither healthcare workers nor spiritual professionals are alone. We share a common quest to enrich the lives of those around us, to create healing and caring environments in the families and communities of those under our care.

No matter how successful we've been in broadening your understanding of spirituality and medicine, you will not be successful in this endeavor if you keep these skills to yourself. So, our final assignment for you is this. Share this book with someone you might collaborate with in caring for others. If you are a physician, discuss this book with a clergy member or a hospital chaplain. If you are a spiritual professional, talk about this book with a physician or other healthcare professional. And, perhaps most importantly, if you ever become a patient, help your physician, your pastor, and your family to talk with one another about your care. Make sure your physician knows about your spiritual values, and talk about your illness and your healthcare with those who care about you. Learning cannot, in the end, succeed if you don't use these skills to create a dialogue. Such a dialogue must begin with someone; we hope that someone is you.

Appendix A

Active listening skills

The true key to the integration of spirituality and medicine is the use of active listening skills. Active listening is necessary for the development of the therapeutic relationship and the development of trust. It is through listening that the clinician can pick up from the patient critical clues that point to a spiritual, emotional, or relational issue. Listening is a functional skill necessary for various interventions. The following descriptions and exercises can be used by clinicians to gain and refine their active listening skills. It can also be used in group settings with clinical staff, medical students or residents to improve their clinical capacity.

Active listening skills all relate back to what is commonly called the 'interpersonal gap.'

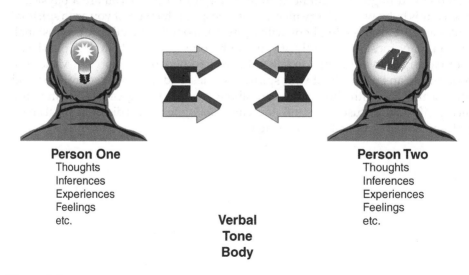

Person One
Thoughts
Inferences
Experiences
Feelings
etc.

**Verbal
Tone
Body**

Person Two
Thoughts
Inferences
Experiences
Feelings
etc.

Figure A.1

When we try to bridge the interpersonal gap we use these codes as a beginning point. However, the task of actually translating them is difficult, and takes work.

Our goal is to learn to use various tools to 'break the code' and do the best job possible of understanding those who are trying to communicate with us.

Blocks to listening
1 The 'How am I doing?' syndrome

This syndrome makes it hard to listen because you're always trying to assess how you are coming across to the person who is talking. 'Am I impressing this person?

Do they like me?' Some people get very competitive here. 'Who is smarter, more competent – me, or the other?' Some people focus on who has suffered more. You can't let much in because you are too busy worrying about how you are doing! This is a particularly tempting problem when you are with a group of new acquaintances.

2 Mind reading

The mind reader doesn't pay much attention to what people say. In fact he/she often distrusts it. This person is trying to figure out what the other person is *really* thinking and feeling. This person also spends a lot of time making assumptions about how people react to you. 'I bet she's looking at my big nose...'

3 Rehearsing/counter story/dreaming

You don't have time to listen when you are rehearsing what you are going to say. Your whole attention is on the preparation and crafting of your next comment. You have to *look* interested, but your mind is going a mile a minute because you have a story to tell, or a point to make. Some people rehearse whole chains of responses. 'I'll say, then he'll say, then I'll say,' and so on. Another version of this is the 'counter story,' where their story brings up a similar episode in your life, that you then 'must' share. At times something the person says suddenly triggers a chain of private associations. Off you go, into your own world.

4 Filtering

When you filter, you listen to some things, and not to others. You pay only enough attention to see if somebody's angry, or unhappy, or if you're in emotional danger. Once assured that the communication contains none of these things, you let your mind wander.

5 Pre-judging

Negative labels have enormous power. If you prejudge someone as stupid or nuts or unqualified, you don't pay much attention to what they say. You've already written them off. A basic rule of listening is that judgments should be made only *after* you have heard and evaluated the content of the message.

6 Advising

You are the great problem solver, ready with help and suggestions. You don't have to hear more than a few sentences before you begin searching for the right advice. However, while you are cooking up suggestions and persuading some to 'just try it,' you may miss what's most important. You didn't hear the feelings, and you didn't acknowledge the person's pain. He or she still feels basically alone because you couldn't listen and just *be* there.

7 Sparring

This block has you arguing and debating with people. The other person never feels heard because you're so quick to disagree. In fact, a lot of your focus is on finding things with which to disagree. You take strong stands, are very clear about your beliefs and preferences. The way to avoid sparring is to repeat back and acknowledge what you've heard. Look for one thing with which you might agree. (One subtype of sparring is the *put-down*. Another type of sparring is discounting. Discounting is for people who can't stand compliments.) Yet another version of this block involves being a person who is 'always right.' Being right means you will go to any lengths (twist the facts, start shouting, make excuses or accusations, call up past sins) to avoid being wrong. You can't listen to criticism, you can't be corrected, and you can't take suggestions to change. Your convictions are unshakable.

8 Derailing

When you derail a conversation, you make comments which block further conversation on that topic. You may change the subject, or joke it off.

9 Placating

'Right... Right... Absolutely... I know... Of course you are... Incredible... Yes... Really?' You want to be nice, pleasant, supportive. You want people to like you. So you agree with everything. You may half-listen, just enough to get the drift, but you're not really involved. You are placating rather than tuning in and examining what's being said.

Identifying blocks

You've read the blocks, and you probably have an idea which ones apply to you. In the space provided, list the blocks that seem typical of the ways to avoid listening.

Assessing your listening blocks

Person	*Blocks*

WORK
   Boss
   Co-workers
   Subordinates

RELATIVES
   Mother
   Father
   Siblings

HOME
   Mate
   Children
   Roommate, etc.

FRIENDS
   Best friend
   Same-sex friends
   Other-sex friends

Look at your pattern of blocking
1   What is your most commonly used block?
2   With whom do you use blocking the most?
3   What subjects or situations usually trigger the block?
4   When you started the block, you were feeling (circle everything that applies)

BORED	ANXIOUS	IRRITATED	HURT	JEALOUS
FRUSTRATED	RUSHED	DOWN	CRITICIZED	EXCITED
PREOCCUPIED	ATTACKED	TIRED	OTHER	_____

The skills for effective listening

- **Paraphrase:** The skill of responding to the content of another person's verbal communication. It identifies with the words by clarifying the content for accuracy. The response should be in your own words, and not a 'parroting' of the content.
- **Perception check:** Responding to the verbal content and the non-verbal messages (through tone and body language) by making a guess as to the feeling or emotion being expressed by the other person.

- **Behavior description:** Describing another person's behavior without making accusations, inferences, and without name calling.
- **Creative questions:** Asking questions based on the free information offered by the other person.
- **Direct expression of feelings:** Naming your own inner emotional state. The ability to identify and name your own inner condition.
- **Fogging:** Stating the truth in another person's critical statement. You affirm only that which is actually true for you.
- **Negative inquiry:** Coaching another person to constructively criticize you in specifics (rather than generalities).

Paraphrase

Definition
Paraphrase is the skill of responding to the content and meaning of another person's verbal communication. It identifies with the *words* by clarifying the content for accuracy.

There are several purposes for a paraphrase:

- to let the other person know you have heard him/her and thus show concern and interest
- to check for accuracy
- to 'buy time'.

Obviously, the more surprising the news or the lengthier the statement, the more important a paraphrase becomes.

Example
- 'It seems to me that our relationship has reached a point of crisis. We no longer talk to one another, we argue incessantly, we have nothing in common, and the feelings of love just aren't present anymore. I think we ought to re-evaluate our relationship.'
  (Paraphrase) 'I hear you saying that our relationship is in real trouble. We don't talk and when we do, we fight. On top of that we don't like to do the same things and you are not sure we love each other anymore. You think perhaps it is time to think about whether we continue to be together.'

Remember, a paraphrase should accurately restate the content of the original statement. It should not infer too much, nor should it try to state the feelings behind the statement.

Perception check

Definition
In a perception check the listener describes what he/she perceives to be the other person's feelings to check for understanding. The goal is to translate the other person's non-verbal communication (gestures, expressions, tone of voice) into a tentative description of feelings. **Remember**, the statement is tentative *and* non-judgmental.

A good perception check conveys this message: 'I want to understand your feelings, is this [description] the way you feel?'

The perception check has four stages.

- **Look and listen:** You listen to the content and look at the non-verbal clues. If there is a clash between the content of the words and the non-verbal behavior, put your trust in the non-verbal message.
- **Think:** You try to identify a feeling. The best way to do this is to get in touch with the feelings the statement stirs up inside you.
- **Share your perception:** Make a tentative statement of what you believe the other person is experiencing.
- **Check:** Ask a question to discover whether your guess was correct. It is not necessary that you always be right. It does help if your guess is close!

Examples
- Verbal: 'Stephen, I want to talk to you about what you said to me this afternoon' (non-verbal: clenched fists, tense throat, voice harsh).
  Check: 'I sense that you are really mad about something I said, am I right?'
- Verbal: 'Steve, I want to talk to you about what you said to me this afternoon' (non-verbal: hands twisting, throat tense, voice harsh, eyes tearing).
  Check: 'I sense that you are really distressed about something, is that true?'

Stems for perception checks
- I get the impression that...
- I'm wondering if...
- It seems to me that...
- It sounds to me as if...
- I have a hunch that...
- It appears to me that...
- Is it possible that you might be feeling...
- I sense that we might have caused you to feel...

If all of this sounds contrived, remember that a perception check is rarely used in isolation from other listening tools.

Example
- 'I am having a terrible time with that specialist you sent me too. We just don't seem to connect and I don't feel like he really cares about me.'
  (Paraphrase) 'So your oncologist and you are having some real problems getting along.'
  (Perception check:) 'I sense that this really has you frustrated. Is that right?'

The goal of a perception check is simple. To move the conversation to a deeper level by giving the speaker permission to tell you how they really feel. Remember, it is not critical that you be absolutely correct. The preceding conversation could end this way:

- 'No, I'm not frustrated, I'm mad! Let me tell you... '

You could block this conversation and not allow your friend to tell you what they need to say. A blocking statement might sound like this:

- 'You think he is bad, you ought to hear some of the stories I have heard about other doctors.'

Exercise
Use the following statements to practice perception checks. Your leader will designate the first person in the sequence. That person will turn to his/her left and say statement 1. Remember to put feeling into the statement through use of tone and body language. What feeling you choose is up to you! The person to the left will respond with a perception check. The rest of the group will monitor the accuracy. After the perception check is completed the person who responded will turn to the person on his/her left and read statement 2, and so on.

1 So, I've got to have surgery, what's next?
2 Doctor, I need to talk to you about my husband/wife...
3 After all that has happened to me, I can no longer believe in God.
4 I have been on this new diet for one month, and I've lost 10 pounds.
5 Let me tell you, this treatment you have me on is really something else...
6 I can't believe how I was treated in the waiting room!

Behavior description
Definition
Behavior description is reporting specific, observable action of other people *without* making accusations, inferences, or name calling. It is a skill that helps the other person become aware of his/her behavior.

Examples
- 'Fran left the meeting 30 minutes early!'
- **Accusation:** Fran is irresponsible.
- **Inference:** Fran was mad.
- 'You interrupted me three times in the last 10 minutes!'
- **Accusation:** You are rude!
- **Inference:** You don't care about me!
- **Name calling:** You jerk!
- 'You are constantly rubbing your hands.'
- **Accusation:** You are weird.
- **Inference:** You are nervous.

Exercise
Read the following statements. Mark a Y for each statement that is a behavior description and an N for each one that is not.

1 ___ The doctor interrupted Jane.
2 ___ Dr Hall is so sincere.
3 ___ Joe was discouraged.
4 ___ Harry's voice got louder when he said, 'that medication isn't helping.'

5 ___ Harry was mad at his doctor.
6 ___ You insulted me!
7 ___ Ann was hurt by Dave's statements.
8 ___ Sue said nothing when Ann said, 'You are a lousy nurse!'
9 ___ Paul talked about the weather and the baseball game.
10 ___ Mark forgot about the meeting.
11 ___ You are inconsiderate!
12 ___ Julie is really mad at Ralph.

Creative questions

Definitions
The ability to ask questions based on 'free' information which will allow the speaker to continue to tell their story.

It is important to note that not all questions are creative. A question is *not* creative if:

- it changes the subject
- it proves too quickly and invades private space
- it is a put-down
- it is 'loaded'
- it can be answered too easily with a 'yes' or 'no.'

It is a creative question if:

- it is congruent and flows naturally from the context of the conversation
- it prompts the other person's story
- it gives the other person permission to say more
- it uses 'free' information given and does not assume knowledge.

Exercise
Here is a statement you might hear when talking to a friend. Assume it is free information in response to one of your questions.

> How am I doing today? I'm really not sure. You know, I used to think I had my life figured out, but some things have happened which have really made me question a lot of things.

1 Write two questions which you think might be facilitating and creative.
2 Write a question that would be blocking or negative.

Direct expression of feeling

Definition
Direct expression of feeling is the act of reporting your own inner feelings as clearly as you can by *directly* expressing those feelings verbally. Direct expression of feeling is sending an 'I' message in which you own your own feelings. It must be understood that many expressions of feeling are indirect.

An indirect expression is offered through:

- body language
- action or behavior

- 'you' statements
- tone of voice
- sarcasm
- etc.

Indirect statements are confusing and often painful. They are to be avoided when at all possible.

Exercise

The following exercise will help you distinguish between direct and indirect statements of feeling. Put a 'D' before all direct statements and an 'I' before all indirect statements.

1 ___ Shut up! Not another word out of you.
2 ___ I'm really angry about what you just said.
3 ___ Can't you see I'm busy, get out!
4 ___ I'm beginning to resent your constant interruptions.
5 ___ I am discouraged by how I am responding to treatment.
6 ___ You don't care about me.
7 ___ You didn't come see me while I was in the hospital.
8 ___ You are a wonderful counselor.
9 ___ I really like you.
10 ___ I feel like I don't understand what you are saying.
11 ___ Everybody likes you.
12 ___ I feel comfortable and free to be myself when I'm around you.
13 ___ I can't believe you would suggest I drink too much!
14 ___ If I don't get better soon, I'm going to find a new doctor.
15 ___ You are a really lousy doctor.
16 ___ I'm confused and frustrated by this news.
17 ___ I feel that we ought to be more open.
18 ___ I will never amount to anything.
19 ___ That doctor is awful, he didn't explain anything.
20 ___ I feel like a failure because I haven't lowered my blood sugar.
21 ___ I feel lonely and alone.
22 ___ I feel as if nobody really cares about me.
23 ___ You slob!!

Responding to criticism

Most of us experience difficulty responding to criticism. The criticism may be directed at us personally, or at an organization or cause we represent. In either case it is difficult not to become defensive, or even offensive. We may find ourselves getting angry in response, we may feel put down, or even guilty.

The difficulty with many of our responses is that they often block communication. A defensive response may well keep us from hearing what the other person has to say and does not allow that person to express and deal with his/her negative feelings.

Even when the criticism appears totally unjustified, we must attempt to keep the communication going. Remember, the feeling is real, whether the conclusions and assumptions are correct or false.

Five kinds of response can be helpful in dealing with criticism. They tend to keep the communication going, let the other person know that he/she is being heard, and help the feelings involved be dealt with. Three of these skills – paraphrase, perception check and direct expression of feeling – we have explored as basic skills. We also introduce two tools specifically focused on difficult exchanges – fogging and negative inquiry.

Paraphrase

This response lets the other person know that you are hearing what he/she has to say and affirms that you heard the statement correctly. It can also help buy time when you need to do some inner processing. Remember, a paraphrase does not analyze, judge, or dig for more – it simply responds to what you hear.

- 'I want to make sure I understand. You are really upset about what your mother has said about your parenting.'

Perception check

This response is useful when the other person is not fully open with his/her feelings. It is a way of responding to non-verbal clues, which in conflict situations are often extensive.

- 'Your tone of voice makes me think you are pretty angry about what I said. Am I right?'

Direct expression of feeling

Another response is to be honest with your own feelings as you hear the other person's criticism. It acknowledges that you too are a person with feelings and it invites a more personal relationship with the other. It is important that your response be direct and that while sharing your own feelings you are also seeking to hear the other.

- 'I want to understand what you are saying, but I am very hurt by your statement and I am struggling with some real anger.'

Fogging

Fogging is agreeing with what is true for you in another person's statement. One of the quickest ways to defuse another's criticism is to agree with the truth in what they are saying. This response is sometimes called 'fogging,' for it is a tactic which simply absorbs the blow, much the way a fog bank simply absorbs all that enters it.

This tactic assumes that there is the possibility of truth in any critical statement. Somewhere! Thus it is important to listen for the element of truth and to agree with it. It is important to note that one does not agree with all that the person says, but only with that part of the statement which has some truth to it.

Examples

    Critic: The doctor never pays me any attention.

    Fogger: You are right, the doctor probably does not interact with you as often as they would like.

    Critic: Doctors just don't care any more.

    Fogger: It is true that many of us find it difficult to show patients the kind of concern that they would desire.

    Critic: All those clinics care about is my money.

    Fogger: You are right, clinics often have to ask patients for payment, and when you are hurting that may feel cold and unfeeling. You must feel as if they don't really care about you (add a perception check). Is that correct?

It is important to note that none of these responses will be sufficient alone. These and other responses must be mixed together for effective communication. It is useful however to separate the various tools for learning and practice.

Negative inquiry

Negative inquiry is the act of coaching the other person in their criticism. Most criticisms begin at a very vague level.

- I don't like you.
- You are a lousy teacher.
- I don't like your hair.

The problem is that these critical statements, being too vague, don't really tell us anything. They are not specific enough to help us understand what the other person doesn't like or wants to change. They certainly don't give us enough information to decide whether the statement is valid and helpful or not.

    We need to help those who are critical of us become more specific in their criticism so we can learn from them, evaluate the statement appropriately, and get to the real issue.

- I hear you saying that you don't like the way I provide you with medical care. What exactly is it that you don't like?

If the person cannot or will not get specific, then you need to be persistent in your attempt to get them to be more helpful.

- I hear your criticism, but I cannot really respond unless you are more specific. Please tell me exactly what it is about my care you do not like.

Continued refusal to be more specific invalidates the criticism. A true criticism can be specific! You can simply refuse to discuss the issue further at that point.

- I am sorry but unless you can be more specific, I really cannot respond.

Giving and receiving feedback

How to give feedback

- Be descriptive: describe specific behaviors.
- Don't use labels: don't use loaded descriptions such as 'unprofessional', 'immature.'
- Don't exaggerate: 'You always ...' 'You never... '
- Don't be judgmental: 'Good,' 'Better,' 'Worse.'
- Speak for yourself: 'Here is *my* feedback.'
- Talk first about yourself: 'I feel,' 'My view...'
- Phrase the issue as a statement.
- Stick to things you know for sure ('just the facts...')
- Help people hear and receive compliments.

A suggested sequence

- Describe the behavior: 'When you...'
- Describe your feelings: 'I feel...'
- Describe how it affects you: 'Because I...'
- Let the other person respond: Pause for discussion ... allow expression.
- Propose a change in behavior: 'I would like...'
- State why you think it will help: 'Because...'
- Listen to the person's response: 'What do you think...' (and really listen!)

When to *avoid* giving feedback

- When you don't know enough about the situation or behavior.
- When you don't care about the person or won't be around to deal with the response.
- When the feedback is about something the person has no power to change.
- When the person's self-esteem is low.
- When your self-esteem is low.
- When your purpose does not have integrity.
- When you want to 'zap' the other person or play some other game.
- When the time and place are not appropriate.

How to receive feedback

- Breathe: It helps manage the stress.
- Listen actively: Don't interrupt, don't jump to the defense.
- Use negative inquiry: Ask for specifics.
- Acknowledge the feedback: Paraphrase! This will give you time to sort things out.
- Acknowledge the valid points: You might even use some fogging here.
- Express your feelings directly: It is OK to let the other person know how this made you feel. It is not OK to dump feelings in an indirect manner!

Appendix B

The Spiritual Involvement and Beliefs Scale

The Spiritual Involvement and Beliefs Scale was developed by RL Hatch, H Spring, L Ritz, and MA Burg from the University of Florida. The Scale in its current 22-question format was revised from an original scale involving 39 questions.

The Scale involves focus on four factors.

Factor	Eigen values	Preliminary factor labels
1	15.0	Core spirituality (connection, meaning, faith, involvement and experience)
2	4.1	Spiritual perspective/existential
3	1.7	Personal application/humility
4	1.2	Acceptance/insight (i.e. insight into futility of focusing attention on things which cannot be changed)

How strongly do you agree with the following statements? Please circle your response. (See opposite.)

	Strongly agree	Agree	Mildly agree	Neutral	Mildly disagree	Disagree	Strongly disagree
1 I set aside time for meditation and/or self-reflection.	7	6	5	4	3	2	1
2 I can find meaning in times of hardship.	7	6	5	4	3	2	1
3 A person can be fulfilled without pursuing an active spiritual life.	7	6	5	4	3	2	1
4 I find serenity by accepting things as they are.	7	6	5	4	3	2	1
5 I have a relationship with someone I can turn to for spiritual guidance.	7	6	5	4	3	2	1
6 Prayers do not really change what happens.	7	6	5	4	3	2	1
7 In times of despair, I can find little reason to hope.	7	6	5	4	3	2	1
8 I have a personal relationship with a power greater than myself.	7	6	5	4	3	2	1
9 I have had a spiritual experience that greatly changed my life.	7	6	5	4	3	2	1
10 When I help others, I expect nothing in return.	7	6	5	4	3	2	1
11 I don't take time to appreciate nature.	7	6	5	4	3	2	1
12 I have joy in my life because of my spirituality.	7	6	5	4	3	2	1
13 My relationship with a higher power helps me love others more completely.	7	6	5	4	3	2	1
14 Spiritual writings enrich my life.	7	6	5	4	3	2	1
15 I have experienced healing after prayer.	7	6	5	4	3	2	1
16 My spiritual understanding continues to grow.	7	6	5	4	3	2	1
17 I focus on what needs to be changed in me, not on what needs to be changed in others.	7	6	5	4	3	2	1
18 In difficult times, I am still grateful.	7	6	5	4	3	2	1
19 I have been through a time of suffering that led to spiritual growth.	7	6	5	4	3	2	1
20 I solve my problems without using spiritual resources.	7	6	5	4	3	2	1
21 I examine my actions to see if they reflect my values.	7	6	5	4	3	2	1
22 How spiritual a person do you consider yourself?	7	6	5	4	3	2	1

Scoring instructions:

Reverse score all **negatively** worded items (3, 6, 7, 11, 20), i.e. Strongly agree = 1, Agree = 2, ... Strongly disagree = 7 or Always = 1, Almost always = 2, ... Never = 7.

Spiritual Involvement and Beliefs Scale – Revised (SIBS-R)

Factors/Questions

Factor 1	Factor 2	Factor 3	Factor 4
1	2	10	4
2	7	17	
3	11		
5	18		
6	21		
8			
9			
12			
13			
14			
15			
16			
18			
19			
20			
22			

Content areas covered on the SIBS-R include:

- Ability to find meaning
- Acceptance
- Application of beliefs and values
- Belief in, connection to, and reliance upon something greater than oneself
- Fulfillment
- Gratitude
- Hope
- Joy
- Love
- Meditation
- Connection to nature
- Prayer
- Relationship between spiritual health and physical health
- Relationship with someone who can provide spiritual guidance
- Serenity

- Service
- Spiritual experiences
- Spiritual growth
- Spiritual writings.

Appendix C

Sample meditations, writing exercises, and drawing exercises

As we noted in Chapter 9, a major tool that can be used to help patients resolve spiritual issues and respond to dis-ease is meditation. There are a variety of types of meditations, and within those types a number of already established meditations. Following are some examples of guided (self-guided, or by tape) meditations that can be used in either the clinical setting, in group settings, or as 'homework.' These meditations come out of the mind/body medicine movement and in some cases are specifically focused on health issues. An excellent resource for those interested in Mind/Body medicine is the Center for Mind-Body Medicine in Washington DC. This organization offers excellent workshops for providers. It is suggested that those interested visit their web site at www.cmbm.org. The Director is Dr James Gordon.

Walking meditation

Purpose
- Tool for developing awareness.
- Good for people who have difficulty with sitting meditation.
- Provides a bridge to help integrate meditative awareness into daily life.

Method
Select a place where you can walk comfortably back and forth, about 30 paces. (In a group setting or in a limited space you can also walk in a circle.) Begin by standing at one end of this 'walking path,' with your feet planted on the ground. Let your hands rest easily, wherever they are comfortable. Close your eyes for a moment, center yourself, and establish the feel of your body standing on the earth. Feel the pressure on the bottoms of your feet and the other natural sensations of standing. Then open your eyes and let yourself be present and alert.

Begin to walk slowly. Let yourself walk with a sense of ease and dignity. Pay attention to your body. With each step, feel the sensations of lifting your foot and leg off the earth. Be aware as you place each foot on the ground. Relax and let your walking be easy and natural. Feel each step mindfully as you walk. You can experiment with the speed, walking at whatever pace keeps you most present. At the end of the path (or at the end of each rotation) pause for a moment and center yourself.

Continue to walk back and forth for 10 or 20 minutes or longer. Your mind will wander away many times. As soon as you notice this, acknowledge where your mind went. You may softly whisper 'wandering,' 'thinking,' 'planning' as a way of noting what has occurred. Then return to the act of feeling the next step. Whether you have been away for one second or for a longer period of time, simply acknowledge where you have been and then come back to being alive here and now with the next step you take.[1]

Body scan meditation

Purpose
- Increases body awareness.
- Can reduce tension, increase calmness and well-being.
- Uses one's own inner wisdom to develop a healing image.

Cautions and contraindications
- May provoke strong emotional memories.

Method/Script
Take a few minutes to get comfortable and to begin to relax. Let yourself shift or move to become more comfortable ... take a few long, slow breaths, and let them go, letting the breath out be a 'letting go' kind of breath. Just let go on each out breath and begin to relax, easily and comfortably, with no effort, just letting yourself begin to focus on the inner world. Just let the outer world 'be.'

When you are ready, see yourself in a protective capsule, just the right size for you, one in which you can see out clearly. Everything you need to be safe and comfortable is available. Now the capsule enters your body in whatever way seems right to you, perhaps through the mouth and stomach into the bloodstream, or on your breath into the lungs and then into the bloodstream. Or perhaps you are just there...

Begin a 'tour' of your body. Perhaps in the abdominal area with the large and small intestines, bladder, liver, spleen, pancreas, stomach, kidneys, and diaphragm. Take a moment to see if there is a place that draws your attention. You may find yourself also going to another part of your body, the chest with heart and lungs, or in your neck or head, thyroid gland, brain ... or in the muscles of your neck, shoulders, and back... Perhaps your attention is drawn to something else not directly physical, such as a relationship, or job, some life problem. That problem could be association with some part of your body, and you can allow your attention to move between the place in your body where you react to that issue and an aspect of the issue itself. Perhaps you are simply curious about your body and stress.

Whatever is happening, wherever you are, move around that place or that issue. What sensations does it have? What is the size, texture, color? As your attention lingers here, what seems to need to happen, what might be helpful? In this mind-body conversation you can begin to consider becoming aware of images, sensations, feelings, concepts, reflecting what could be helpful to you. It could be anything. As you listen, your inner wisdom can be heard in a quiet way.

Now prepare to take your leave, promising yourself to return and continue the process of self-discovery and healing. Bring yourself back to this place and time at your own pace.

---

[1] Adapted from Kornfield J (1993) *A Path with Heart: a guide through the perils and promises of spiritual life*. Bantam Books, New York, NY, pp.66–7.

Forgiveness meditation

Purpose
- Can help make peace with the past.
- Foster connection rather than isolation.
- Can facilitate profound emotional healing.

Cautions and contraindications
- May provoke strong emotional memories.

Meditation script
Close your eyes, relax, and bring your attention to your breath. Bring awareness to the in-breath and to the out-breath. Let the breath help you let go, let yourself float in a great heart, resting. Bring up an image of someone for whom you have anger or resentment. Let yourself see that person now. Choose whomever you like. It doesn't have to be the person who has hurt you the most, just someone for whom you hold resentment. Invite that person into your heart, just for a moment. Look that person in the eye and say to them, 'I forgive you.' Soften toward that person. Let them linger in your heart just for now. Now bid them farewell. 'I forgive you.'

Return to your breath, resting in the circle of creation. Breathing in, you know you are breathing in. Breathing out, you know you are breathing out. Now invite into your heart someone whom you have harmed in some way. Invite them in and say: 'Forgive me. For whatever I may have done to harm you, forgive me.' Open your heart to theirs, and swell, for the moment, in the same circle. Resting, softening, in forgiveness. Following your breath. Breathing in, breathing out, forgiveness. And now bid them farewell.

Now invite yourself into you heart. Look at yourself, surrounded by the loving kindness of your heart. And say to yourself, 'I forgive you.' For whatever you feel you have done to hurt yourself, for however you have let yourself down. 'I forgive you.' Let the sensation of softening expand. Let the forgiveness expand to fill the entire planet. All the beings in need of forgiveness. 'I forgive you.'[2]

Writing exercise/meditation: 'dialogue with a symptom'

Purpose
- Tool for self-awareness.
- Helps access subconscious information about a problem or symptom.
- Strengthens awareness of inner wisdom.

Cautions and contraindications
- May provoke strong emotional memories.

---

[2] Adapted from Levine S (1987) *Healing into Life and Death*. Anchor Press, Garden City, NY.

Method

- Relax and center for three to five minutes.
- Think of your symptom or problem as if it were a person with its own separate history. Recall this history and write it down if you like. For example: When was the symptom 'born'? What have been the high and low points in its life? When does it come to visit or seek attention?
- When you have finished, rest with your eyes closed for a few minutes.
- Imagine the symptom or problem sitting in the chair across the room from you. Name it if you like. Write, as fast as you can, without edition and without rereading a conversation between yourself and the symptom or problem. Continue writing until you feel complete. When you are finished, reread what you've written.[3]

Drawing exercise

Normally a group exercise, to be used at the beginning and end of a set of sessions. Can be used with an individual at the beginning and end of a set of sessions.

Materials

- Drawing paper.
- Crayons.

Purpose

- Tool for self-awareness.
- Helps individual or group members to access unconscious information.
- Provides 'before' and 'after' information, a way to evaluate changes.

Cautions and contraindications

- May provoke strong emotions.

Method

A   First set of drawings (session one)
1 Draw:
yourself as you are right now
yourself with your biggest problem
yourself as you'd like to be.
2 After the drawings are completed the group facilitator or the clinician collects the drawing(s) and keeps them until the final session.
B   Closing set of drawings (final session)
1 Draw:
yourself as you are now
yourself as you'd like to be
how you are going to get there.
2 Facilitator or clinician returns the first set of drawings to each person, and each person compares his/her two sets.

---

[3] Adapted from Travis J and Ryan RS (1988) *Wellness Workbook*. Ten Speed Press, Berkeley, CA, p.13.

Appendix D

Suggested further reading

General reading

Benson H (1997) *Timeless Healing: the power and biology of belief.* Fireside Books (Simon & Schuster), New York, NY.

Faiver C, Ingersoll RE, O'Brien E and McNally C (2001) *Explorations in Counseling and Spirituality.* Thomson Learning – Brooks/Cole, Belmont, CA.

Gallup G Jr and Lindsay MD (1999) *Surveying the Religious Landscape.* Morehouse Publishing, Harrisburg, PA.

Gordon JS (1996) *Manifesto for a New Medicine.* Addison-Wesley, Reading, MA, pp.17–18.

King DE (2000) *Faith, Spirituality, and Medicine.* Haworth Pastoral Press, New York, NY.

Koenig H (1997) *Is Religion Good for Your Health?* Haworth Pastoral Press, New York, NY.

Koenig H (2001) *The Healing Power of Faith.* Touchstone Books, New York, NY.

Koenig HG, McCullough ME and Larson DB (2001) *Handbook of Religion and Health.* Oxford University Press, New York, NY.

Matthews D (1998) *The Faith Factor.* Viking, New York, NY.

Miller WR (ed.) (1999) *Integrating Spirituality into Treatment.* American Psychological Association, Washington DC.

Numbers RL and Amundsen DW (eds) (1986) *Caring and Curing.* The Johns Hopkins University Press, Baltimore, MD.

Myss C (1996) *Anatomy of the Spirit.* Three Rivers Press, New York.

Propst LR (1988) *Psychotherapy in a Religious Framework.* Human Sciences Press, New York, NY.

Steward M, Brown JB, Weston WW, McWhinney IR, McWilliam CL and Freeman TR (2003) *Patient Centered Medicine: transforming the clinical method* (2e). Radcliffe Medical Press, Oxford.

Integration into the exam room

Anadarajah G and Hight E (2001) Spirituality and medical practice: using the HOPE questions as a practical tool for spiritual assessment. *American Family Physician.* 63(January 1): 1.

Benson H (1997) *Timeless Healing: the power and biology of belief.* Fireside Books (Simon & Schuster), New York, NY.

Bryant-Jefferies R (2003) *Time Limited Therapy in Primary Care.* Radcliffe Medical Press, Oxford.

Daaleman TP and Frey B (1998) Prevalence and patterns of physician referral to clergy and pastoral care providers. *Arch Fam Med.* 7: 548–53.

Ehman JW, Ott BB and Short TH (1999) Do patients want physicians to inquire about their spiritual or religious beliefs if they become gravely ill? *Arch Intern Med.* 159(15): 1803–6.

Hirsh SK and Kise JAG (1998) *Soul Types*. Hyperion Press, New York, NY.

Hodges S (1999) Spiritual screening: the starting place for intentional pastoral care. *Chaplaincy Today*. **15**(1): 30–9.

Kristeller JL and Rhodes M (2002) The OASIS Project: oncologist-assisted spirituality intervention study. Presented at *Spirituality and Health Care*, Salt Lake City, UT, March.

Larson DB, Swyers JP and McCullough ME (1997) *Scientific Research on Spirituality and Health: a consensus report*. National Institute for Healthcare Research, Rockville, MD.

Levinson W, Gorawara-Bhat R and Lamb J (2000) A study of patient clues and physician responses in primary care and surgical settings. *JAMA*. **284**(8): 1021–7.

Maugans TA (1996) The spiritual history. *Arch Fam Med*. **5**(Jan): 11–16 (SPIRIT Model).

Pulchalski CM and Romer AL (2000) Taking a spiritual history allows clinicians to understand patients more fully. *Journal of Palliative Medicine*. **3**: 129–37.

Thiel MM and Robinson MR (1997) Physicians' collaboration with chaplains: difficulties and benefits. *Journal of Clinical Ethics*. **8**(1): 94–103.

Ussivakul AV (2003) *An Introduction to Buddhist Meditation for Results*. Tippayawisuit Ltd Partnership, Bangkok, Thailand. (For information contact Sally Timm at istimm@pacifier.com.)

Walker L (2002) *Consulting with NLP: neuro-linguistic programming in the medical consultation*. Radcliffe Medical Press, Oxford.

Specific issues

The clinician's own spirituality

Daaleman TP and Frey B (1999) Spiritual and religious beliefs and practices of family physicians: a national survey. *J Fam Pract*. **48**(2): 98–104.

Graiagie F and Hobbs R III (1999) Spiritual perspectives and practices of family physicians with an expressed interest in spirituality. *Fam Med*. **31**(8): 578–85.

Maugans TA and Wadland WC (1991) Religion and family medicine: a survey of physicians and patients. *J Fam Pract*. **32**(2): 210–13.

Patient spirituality

Daaleman TP and Nease DE Jr (1994) Patient attitudes regarding physician inquiry into spiritual and religious issues. *J Fam Pract*. **39**: 564–8.

Seidel HM, Ball JW, Dains JE and Benedict GW (1995) *Mosby's Guide to Physical Examination* (3e). Mosby, St Louis, MO.

Veatch RM (ed.) (1989) *Cross Cultural Perspectives in Medical Ethics: readings*. Jones and Bartlett, Boston. Selected articles, start pp.44, 58, 120, 126, 130, 132, 140.

Issues and roadblocks

Ellis M, Vinson D and Ewigman B (1999) Addressing spiritual concerns with patients: family physicians attitudes and practices. *J Fam Pract*. **48**(2): 105–9.

Post SG, Puchalski CM and Larson DB (2000) Physicians and patient spirituality: professional boundaries, competency, and ethics. *Annals of Internal Medicine*. **132**(7): 578–83.

Sloan RP, Bagiella E, VandeCreek L *et al*. (2000) Should physicians prescribe religious activities? *N Engl J Med*. **342**: 1913–16 (Sounding Board).

Sloan RP, Bagiella E and Powell T (1999) Religion, spirituality, and medicine. *The Lancet*. **353**: 664–7.

Spirituality in specific situations

Arnold JC (1996) *I Tell You a Mystery*. The Plough Publishing House, Farmington, PA, pp.122–7.

Albertson SH (1980) *Endings and Beginnings*. Ballantine, NY.

Carroll S (1993) Spirituality and purpose in life in alcoholism recovery. *Journal of Studies on Alcohol*. **54**(3): 297–301.

Derrickson BS (1996) The spiritual work of the dying: a framework and case studies. *The Hospice Journal*. **11**(2): 11–30.

Kubler Ross E (1969) *On Death and Dying*. Macmillan, NY.

Index

A-B-C-D-E system, spiritual interventions
  177–9
abandonment 114–15
abortion experience 172
Agnes
  amplification experience 114–15
  cancer experience 80, 114–15
agnostic, personal spirituality 106
Al, self-awareness experience 111–12
amplification, integration objective 113–15
Andrea, communication experience 87–8
anger 67–8
  projected 169
anger experience, Peter 169
anger–forgiveness 76–8
Ann
  sexual abuse 48
  spiritual experience 48
Anne
  car accident experience 120
  options creation 120
  sexual abuse 161–5
'anti-goals,' integration objective 123–4
anxiety 59–61, 63–5
  defining 63–4
  types 59–60
application, spirituality 35–8, 61
assessment, spiritual *see* spiritual assessment
audio characteristics, neuro-linguistics 94–7
awareness creation, spiritual interventions
  172–5
awareness, self-awareness 110–13

Bacon, Francis 25–6
Baha'i, personal spirituality 105
barriers, integration 33
behavior description, listening 140–1, 198–9
belief domain, spirituality 47–8
beliefs, troubling 156–9
Ben, guilt 70–1
Bob, body language 173
body language
  Bob 173
  communication 85, 128–9
  information, gathering 173
body, personhood 10–12
boundaries, integration 39–42

The Brothers Karamazov 37
Buddhism 5–6
  Nirvana 5–6
  Noble Truths 5–6
Byrd study 35

calculators, personal culture 92, 93
cancer experiences
  Agnes 80, 114–15
  Carl 119
  David 51–4
  May 75
  Paul 20–2
car accident experience, Anne 120
Carl
  cancer experience 119
  options creation 119
Catholic, personal spirituality 103–4
challengers, personal culture 92–3
change stimulation, spiritual interventions
  175–9, 180–5
changes, spiritual/religious 154–6
chaplains 109–10, 185–6
Charlie, anger–forgiveness 77
chasm, integration 24–8
child, death of 56
Christian, personal spirituality 105
clinical encounter, multifaceted 133
coherence
  health 2, 18
  life 18–19
collaborative interventions 185–8
colon cancer experience, May 75
communication 84–9
  see also information gathering; listening
  body language 85, 128–9
  cultures 84–9
  indirect statements 128–9
  neuro-linguistics 94–7
  process 84–9
  protective 128–33
  stories 129–30
The Confusion of Modern Man 7–9
connected–disconnected 81
consequential dimension, spirituality
  47
corrective self 69

counseling 167
 spiritual counselors 186
creative questions, listening 141, 199
criticism, responding to 200–2
cultures
 communication 84–9
 culture of one 84–108
 internal factors 93–7
 personal 89–93
 spiritual 97–100
cures, and healing 20–2

dark side, spirituality 65–8
David, cancer experience 51–4
de Rougemont, Dr Jean 7
definitions, personhood 6–9
depression, Mr R 66
Descartes 24–45
despair–hope 74–5
dimensions, spirituality 47–54
direct expression of feeling
 criticism 201
 listening 199–200
dis-ease 3
 sense of 63
 spiritual 72–3
disconnected–connected 81
disruption, spirituality relationship 58–61
domains
 domain-focused case scenarios 52–3
 health 2–3
 spirituality 47–54
Dostoevsky 37
drawing exercise 211

Ellis, Albert 72–3
emotional healing 130–3
empathy
 integration objective 121–3
 trust 171–2
empathy experience, Neil 172
empowerment–helplessness 75–6
environmental factors, personal cultures 90–3
existential anxiety 59–60
experience domain, spirituality 47–8
experiential dimension, spirituality 47
exploring spirituality 46–62

faith systems, personhood in 3–6
fear/discontent–serenity 79–81
feedback, giving/receiving 203
filters, universal, spiritual assessment 152–3
fogging, listening 201–2

forgiveness–anger 76–8
fragmentation of life 18–19
Frameworks 18–19

groups, support/study 187–8
growth stimulation, spiritual interventions
  180–5
guilt 69–71, 111–12, 166
guilt–restoration 78–9

Harvey, lung condition experience 10–12
healing
 and cures 20–2
 and health 17–22
 whole person 1–23
health
 coherence 2, 18
 defining 18
 and healing 17–22
health domains 2–3
health outcomes, spirituality 30–2
helplessness–empowerment 75–6
Hindu, personal spirituality 105
hope–despair 74–5
hopelessness/helplessness 65–7
Howard, Parkinson's disease experience 56
humanistic spirituality 14

ideal self 69
identity, pianist's experience 1
ideological dimension, spirituality 47
impact, spirituality 63–83
impetus
 from patient need 32
 from research 28–32
independence loss, Mr B 65
information gathering 126–46
 see also communication; listening
 body language 173
 indirect statements 128–9
 issue related clues 130–3
 listening 131–42
 multifaceted approach 126–7
 spiritual interventions 172–5
 stories 129–30
 tools 143–5
 whole person 126–7
integration
 amplification 113–15
 'anti-goals' 123–4
 barriers 33
 boundaries 39–42
 chasm 24–8

empathy   121–3
  implications   89
  key issues   34–42
  model   24–45
  objectives   109–25
  options creation   118–21
  patient need   32
  point, counter-point   33–4
  reframing   115–18
  research   28–32
  self-awareness   110–13
  spirituality use/misuse   35–8
  support   121–3
intellectual dimension, spirituality   47
internal factors   93–7
interventions, spiritual *see* spiritual interventions
inventories, spiritual   159–61
irrational ideas   176–7

John, guilt   166
journey, spirituality as   54–7
Jude, reframing experience   116

key issues, integration   34–42
kinesthetic characteristics, neuro-linguistics
        94–7

Laennec   1–2
language of healing   134–42
limitations, spiritual interventions   167–8
listening   192–200
  see also communication; information gathering
  behavior description   140–1, 198–9
  blocks   134–7, 192–5
  communication   131–42
  creative questions   141, 199
  direct expression of feeling   199–200
  fogging   201–2
  negative inquiry   141–2, 202
  paraphrasing   137–8, 196
  perception check   138–40, 196–8
  skills   137–42, 195–200
  trust   171–2
loss   129–30
lung condition experience, Harvey   10–12
Lutheran, personal spirituality   106
lymphoma experience, Carl   119

Martha, communication experience   87–8
May, colon cancer experience   75
MBTI *see* Myers-Briggs Type Indicator
meaninglessness   71–2
medicine, and spirituality   24–8

meditation   182–4
  samples   208–11
mesothelioma experience, Paul   20–2
Myers-Briggs Type Indicator (MBTI)   94
Miller, William   2
mind-body medicine   186–7
moored spirituality   14–15
moral anxiety   59–60
Mr B, independence loss   65
Mr P, spinal cord injury   68
Mr R
  depression   66
  weight problem   66
multifaceted approach, gathering
        information   126–7
multifaceted clinical encounter   133
Muslim, personal spirituality   101–3
Myss, Caroline   37–8

neck pain, body language   173
negative inquiry, listening   141–2, 202
Neil, empathy experience   172
neuro-linguistics   94–7, 152–3
neurotic anxiety   59–60
Nirvana, Buddhism   5–6
Noble Truths, Buddhism   5–6

obesity experiences   66, 111–12
options creation, integration objective   118–21
outcomes, health, spirituality   30–2

pancreatic cancer experience
  Agnes   80
  David   51–4
paraphrasing
  criticism   201
  listening   137–8, 196
  spiritual assessment   150
Parkinson's disease experience, Howard   56
patient need, impetus from   32
Paul, cancer experience   20–2
Peoplemaking   9
perception check
  criticism   201
  listening   138–40, 196–8
person, defined   10–12
personal cultures   89–93
  environmental factors   90–3
personal spirituality   101–7
  Roman Catholic   103–4
personhood
  body   10–12
  definitions   6–9

in faith systems 3–6
  philosophical definitions 6–9
  psychological definitions 6–9
  psychotherapy 9
  self 10–12
  social self 10–12
  soul 10–12
  spiritual self 10–12
  triangle model 7–9
Peter, anger experience 169
philosophical definitions, personhood 6–9
physical outcomes, spirituality 31
pianist's experience, identity 1
postal worker, independence loss 65
power, integration barrier 39–40
practice domain, spirituality 47–8
prayer 35–6, 47, 102–3, 132, 184–5
  Serenity Prayer 79
psychological definitions, personhood 6–9
psychotherapy, personhood 9
punitive self 69–71

real anxiety 59–60
reconciliation 77–8
reflection stimulation, spiritual
    interventions 175–9
reframing, integration objective 115–18
relationship, spirituality as 57–61
relaxation techniques 180–1
religion
  characteristics 12, 16
  impact 72–3
  personal spirituality 101–7
  and science 24–8
religious beliefs 98–100
religious changes 154–6
religious leaders 186
religious orientation 154–6
research
  areas 30
  impetus from 28–32
  integration 28–32
  quality 34–5
  spirituality 28–32
resource, spirituality as 73–82
responsibility 37
restoration–guilt 78–9
ritualistic dimension, spirituality 47
Roman Catholic, personal spirituality 103–4
de Rougemont, Dr Jean 7

Satir, Virginia 9
science, and religion 24–8

self
  personhood 10–12
  types 69–71
self-awareness, integration objective 110–13
serenity, characteristics 79–80
serenity–fear/discontent 79–81
Serenity Prayer 79
Seventh Day Adventist, personal
    spirituality 105
sexual abuse
  Ann 48
  Anne 161–5
Shirley
  helplessness–empowerment 76
  spiritual experience 48–9
SIBS *see* Spiritual Involvement and Beliefs Scale
social self, personhood 10–12
soul 4–5
  personhood 10–12
spectrum, spiritual issues spectrum 73–82,
    161–5
spinal cord injury, Mr P 68
Spirit 4–5
spiritual assessment 147–65
  context 147–51
  paraphrasing 150
  religious changes 154–6
  spiritual changes 154–6
  spiritual inventories 159–61
  tools 151–3
  troubling beliefs 156–9
  universal filters 152–3
spiritual changes 154–6
spiritual counselors 186
spiritual cultures 97–100
spiritual distress/dis-ease, impact 72–3
spiritual exercises 181–2
spiritual experiences 48–9
  Ann 48
  domain 48–9
  Shirley 48–9
spiritual inquiry, tools 143–5
spiritual interventions 166–90
  A-B-C-D-E system 177–9
  awareness creation 172–5
  categories 170–1
  change stimulation 175–9, 180–5
  collaborative interventions 185–8
  growth stimulation 180–5
  information, gathering 172–5
  limitations 167–8
  preparing for 167–71
  prerequisites 169–70

reflection stimulation   175–9
trust   171–2
understanding levels   167
use of   171–88
spiritual inventories   159–61
Spiritual Involvement and Beliefs Scale
        (SIBS)   204–7
spiritual issues spectrum   73–82, 161–5
spiritual, realm of   12–17
spiritual self, personhood   10–12
spiritual themes, expression   131
spirituality
    application   35–8, 61
    dark side   65–8
    defining   13
    dimensions   47–54
    domains   47–54
    exploring   46–62
    health outcomes   30–2
    impact   63–83
    as journey   54–7
    and medicine   24–8
    personal   101–7
    physical outcomes   31
    as relationship   57–61
    research   28–32
    as resource   73–82
    stages   37–8
    types   14–15
    use/misuse   35–8
stages, spirituality   37–8
stereotyping   89
Stocker, Alex   7–9
stories, communication   129–30
strivers, personal culture   91–2

study groups   187–8
suggested reading   212–14
support groups   187–8
support, integration objective   121–3
supportive dimension, spirituality   47

technology   19
temperament   94
time issues, integration barrier   40–1
tools
    spiritual assessment   151–3
    spiritual inquiry   143–5
Tournier, Paul   6–9
training, integration barrier   41–2
triangle model, personhood   7–9
troubling beliefs, spiritual assessment
        156–9
trust, spiritual interventions   171–2

Unitarian-Universalist, personal
        spirituality   105, 106
universal filters, spiritual assessment   152–3
unmoored spirituality   14
use/misuse, spirituality   35–8

visual characteristics, neuro-linguistics   94–7

Walrath, DA   18–19
weight problem
    Al   111–12
    Mr R   66
whole person   1–23
    gathering information   126–7
The Whole Person in a Broken World   6–7
writing exercise   210–11